TABLE OF CONTENTS

TABLE OF CONTENTS 3

CHAPTER 1: BASIC NATIVE AMERICAN PRINCIPLES AND APPROACH TO HEALING, GOOD HEALTH AND WELLNESS 31

The guiding principles of the Native American healing process 31

Healing and wellness are holistic 36

Healing and wellness are herbalistic 36

Cleanliness is connected to good health and dirtiness is connected to disease 37

Healing and wellness are naturalistic and safe, yet effective 37

The body is sacred and food is medicine 38

CHAPTER 2: NATIVE AMERICAN HERBS AND MEDICINAL PLANTS AND THEIR SPECIFIC USES IN THE HEALING OF DIFFERENT DISEASES AND CONDITIONS 40

CHAPTER 3: THE LEADING DISEASE-CAUSES OF DEATH IN THE USA AND THEIR NATIVE-AMERICAN HERBAL CURES AND REMEDIES 93

HEART DISEASE **93**

Hawthorn berry 93

Sassafras 94

Sweetflag or calamus 94

NATIVE AMERICAN HERBALISM

MEDICINAL PLANTS & HERBAL REMEDIES HANDBOOK

Natural Remedies to Heal Major Diseases and Common Ailments

BY

RICHARD B. HORSENECK

COPYRIGHT

DISCLAIMER

The information given and opinions expressed in this book, publication are for informational and educational purposes only and do not replace medical advice or constitute the practice of medicine in any way, shape or form. No doctor-patient, provider-patient, professional-client or provider-client relationship (whether explicit or implicit) exists or has been created between the authors and publishers of this book, publication and the readers or any specific reader.

Many of the strategies discussed in this book, publication may be less effective than proven, modern-day medications, pharmaceuticals and medical technology. Also the herbs, plants, ingredients, products and items, etc. mentioned in this book may contain potent chemical compounds that can be dangerous if not used properly. Therefore, the authors and publishers of this book, publication strongly admonish the readers or any specific reader to always seek standard, professional and modern medical consultation, advice and services from certified and licensed medical practitioners and to take, use, apply, consume or ingest any herbs, plants, ingredients, products and items, etc. mentioned or cited in this book, only under the approval, prescription, supervision and guidance of a licensed medical practitioner.

The reader and any and all specific readers should never delay to seek medical advice and/or disregard medical advice

American hemp, dogbane 94

Purslane 94

Rosehips 95

White willow.............................95

Red clover 95

Violet Prairieclover 95

CANCER......................96

Creosote bush 96

Greater Burdock 97

Greater celandine..................98

Cancer root............................98

Cancer weed 99

Western larch 99

Indian pokeroot......................99

Bloodroot 99

White willow 99

Sheep sorrel 100

Goldenseal........................... 100

Chishima zasa 100

Desert thorn 100

Hound's tongue.................... 100

Akebia 100

CHRONIC LOWER RESPIRATORY DISEASES (CHRONIC BRONCHITIS, EMPHYSEMA AND ASTHMA)

.... 101

Common Yarrow.................. 103

Brewer's Angelica 103

Forked Sagewort 103

Big Sagebrush 103

Curlycup Gumweed.............104

Carrotleaf Biscuitroot...........104

Indian Walnut 104

Indianhemp.........................104

American Spikenard.............104

Stinking Chamomile 104

Horseradish 104

Licorice Bedstraw................104

Cultivated Licorice...............104

Man of The Earth 104

Meadow Garlic 104

Cultivated Garlic..................104

Wild Garlic..........................105

Hyssop 105

Elecampane Inula 105

Oahu Wormwood 105

Olapa 105

Elecampane Inula 105

California Sycamore 106

Grand Fir..................... 106

Subalpine Fir................. 106

Calamus...................... 106

Red Baneberry................. 106

White Colicroot 106

Scarlet Indian Paintbrush..... 107

STROKE AND CEREBROVASCULAR DISEASES 107

White willow 107

Bilberry..................... 107

Anti-high blood pressure herbal group 108

Anti-cholesterol, anti-blood clotting, anti-stroke herbal group 108

Annual Ragweed 108

Wild Strawberry 109

Western Pearlyeverlasting ...109

Elecampane Inula 109

American Skunkcabbage 109

ALZHEIMER'S DISEASE .109

Celery seeds 111

Rosemary 111

Turmeric 112

Greater burdock 113

American ginseng 113

Beggarslice 113

Mediterranean diet 113

Lemon balm 115

Person-centric care 115

Preventing Alzheimer's disease 116

DIABETES 116

Calamus 117

Yerba Mansa 117

Wild Sarsaparilla 117

American Spikenard 117

Pacific Madrone 118

Horseradish 118

Alaska Sagebrush 118

Boreal Sagebrush 118

Fringed Sagewort.................118

New Jersey tea....................118

Sweet woodreed 118

Yellowspine Thistle 118

Yellow Bluebeadlily 118

Pink lady's slipper................119

Lesser yellow lady's slipper..119

Queen Anne's lace 119

Spurge................................119

Rocky Mountain Juniper.......119

Oregon Bitterroot.................119

Devilsclub 119

Nightblooming Cereus..........120

Common Selfheal.................120

Sumac 120

Evergreen Huckleberry 120

Frost Grape 120

Adam's Needle 120

Sage 121

Brazilian Orchid Tree 121

Pfaffia 121

Prevention of diabetes 121

INFLUENZA AND PNEUMONIA

.... **122**

Wild Sarsaparilla 122

Big Sagebrush 123

Summer Coralroot 123

Curlycup Gumweed 123

Common Hop 123

Western Juniper 124

Rocky Mountain Juniper......124

Juniper Wood.....................124

Carrotleaf Biscuitroot..........124

Western Sweetroot 124

Common Yarrow 125

Foothill Sagewort 125

Butterfly Milkweed..............125

Tasselflower Brickellbush 125

Fendler's Bedstraw..............125

Common Hop.....................125

Oceanspray........................125

Horehound 125

Sharpleaf Valerian...............125

Nevada Smokebush..............125

Hairy Horsebrush.................126

Lodgepole Pine 126

Bud Sagebrush 126

KIDNEY DISEASE 126

Balsam Fir........................... 127

Striped Maple...................... 127

Common Yarrow.................. 127

Western Yarrow 127

Black Bugbane..................... 128

Indianhemp 128

Drummond's Rockcress....... 128

Kinnikinnick........................ 128

Milkweed 129

Pipsissewa 129

Watermelon 129

Devil's Darning Needles 129

Squash 130

Prevention of kidney disease 130

SEPTICEMIA 130

Annual Ragweed 131

American Spikenard 131

Tilesius' Wormwood 131

Sacred Thornapple 131

Redroot Buckwheat 131

Idaho Hymenopappus 132

Harlequin Blueflag 132

American Skunkcabbage 132

Starry False Solomon's Seal 132

White Spruce 132

Pin Cherry 132

Red Oak 132

Blue Elderberry 133

European Red Elderberry 133

California False Hellebore ... 133

Prevention of septicemia 133

CHRONIC LIVER DISEASE 133

Watercress 135

Common Yarrow 135

Northern Maidenhair 135

Spreading Dogbane 135

American Spikenard 135

Horseflyweed 136

Common Barberry 136

Yellow Birch 136

Nodding Onion 136

Maidenhair Spleenwort 136

Sharplobe Hepatica..............136

Dwarf Crested Iris.................136

Dwarf Violet Iris 136

Virginia Iris..........................136

Purple Passionflower 136

Summer Grape.....................136

Fox Grape 136

Frost Grape 137

Indian Physic.......................137

Bowman's Root 137

Culver's Root.......................137

Mockernut Hickory 137

Shellbark Hickory 137

Sand Hickory 137

White Colicroot....................137

Virginia Strawberry 137

Virginia Creeper 137

Mountain Sweetpepperbush 137

Common Persimmon 137

Wild Hydrangea 137

Ashy Hydrangea 137

False Aloe 137

Dwarf Ginseng 137

Prevention of liver disease and cirrhosis 137

HIV 138

Creosote bush 138

Carqueja 138

Moreton Bay Chestnut 139

OBESITY 140

Woolly Plantain.....................140

Colorado four o'clock...........140

Snowbrush 140

Chamisso's Manfern............140

Male Fern 140

Oregon Crabapple...............140

Buckthorn 141

Yerba Mate.......................141

Stevia 141

CHAPTER 4: SPECIFIC DISEASES AND CONDITIONS AND THEIR NATIVE AMERICAN HERBAL CURES AND REMEDIES 142

Asthma 142

Backache..........................142

Bronchitis.........................143

Burns.................................. 144

Childbirth (for a quick delivery)
.... 144

Colds................................... 146

Colic................................... 146

Contraceptives..................... 146

Coughs................................ 148

Diabetes.............................. 148

Diarrhea 149

Fevers 151

Headache 152

Heart and circulatory problems
.... 153

Hemorrhoids 154

Herpes zoster (shingles)...... 154

Indigestion 155

Inflammations and swellings 155

Influenza 156

Insect bites and stings 157

Insect repellents, insecticides 160

Rheumatism 163

Sedatives 165

Skin conditions 167

Thrush 170

Yeast infections 171

CHAPTER 5: THE MOST-
IMPORTANT HERBS THAT NATIVE
AMERICANS USED EVERYDAY TO
CURE EVERYTHING 173

Ashwagandha 174

Blackberry 174

Black gum bark 175

Buckbrush 175

Cattail................................. 175

Curly dock 177

Devil's claw 178

Geranium 178

Greenbriar.......................... 179

Honeysuckle 179

Lavender 179

Licorice root 179

Mint 180

Mullein................................ 181

Prickly pear cactus............. 182

Rose hip.............................. 182

Rosemary............................ 183

Sage.................................... 183

Sumac 185

Uva ursi 186

Valerian 186

Wild black cherry 187

Wild ginger 187

Wild rose 188

Witch hazel 189

Yarrow 189

CHAPTER 6: NATIVE AMERICAN HERBAL CURES AND REMEDIES FOR DENTAL HEALTH 190

Antimicrobials for oral health 190

Toothaches......................... 191

Swelling and bleeding 199

Aphthous ulcers 205

Sore throats....................... 206

Periodontal disease, caries and inflammation 210

CHAPTER 7: NATIVE AMERICAN HERBAL SECRETS FOR BEAUTY AND PERSONAL CARE 213

PERSONAL HYGIENE: THE SECRETS OF COLD WATER 213

The benefits of cold water.... 213

SKIN ISSUES................ 213

For faster wound healing, hydrating the skin, soothing itches and irritation and soothing sunburn 213

For moisturizing and softening the skin and for healing skin conditions.......................... 214

For repairing and restoring
mature or damaged skin 214

Natural sunscreen 214

Protect lips from the elements215

Skin cancer.........................215

If you get sunburned anyway215

For skin dryness, rashes,
breakouts and eczema........215

For oily or dirty skin 215

For tightening facial skin pores
and a glowing face 216

For detoxifying the skin 216

For removal of oil, dirt, impurities
and the opening of facial skin
pores 216

For poison ivy, bites and rashes.
....216

For warts 216

For acne............................. 217

Teeth care.......................... 217

Natural toothbrush/ tooth scrubber 217

Natural toothpick.................. 217

HAIR CARE/ HAIR ISSUES

.... **217**

Best water for washing hair . 217

For faster hair growth.......... 217

For incredibly shiny hair....... 218

For repairing and restoring mature or damaged hair 218

For moisturizing, softening hair 218

For well-moisturized, shiny hair
...................................218

For healthy, thick and strong hair
...................................218

For eliminating hair lice 219

For eliminating gray hair......219

Baldness cure – for growing your
hair back..............................219

COSMETICS 219

Rouge and face lifter 219

Eye-brow care 220

MANAGING SMELLS 220

Creating nice smells.............220

Masking foot odor.................220

Masking body odor...............221

Masking mouth odor.............221

LONGEVITY **221**

How to stay young despite your age 221

CHAPTER 8: NATIVE AMERICAN HERBAL SECRETS FOR LOVE, PASSION, FLIRTING, APHRODISIACS, GETTING PREGNANT OR BUILDING A LONG-LASTING MARRIAGE 222

For flirting and attracting love222

Aphrodisiacs 222

For reversing impotence 226

For getting pregnant 226

For preventing pregnancy (contraceptive) 227

For broken hearts 229

For a stable and long-lasting marriage 229

CHAPTER 9: SPECIAL NATIVE AMERICAN HERBAL REMEDIES FOR MAKING YOURSELF FLU-PROOF 232

CHAPTER 10: HOW TO HANDLE. PREPARE AND STORE HERBS FOR GOOD HEALTH AND WELLNESS237

Harvesting 239

Drying 239

Preparing.................................240

Teas and infusions 241

Decoctions............................241

Poultices................................242

Herbal remedies and children243

Additional guidelines for gathering 243

Additional guidelines for drying 244

Storing............................... 245

CHAPTER 1: BASIC NATIVE AMERICAN PRINCIPLES AND APPROACH TO HEALING, GOOD HEALTH AND WELLNESS

The guiding principles of the Native American healing process

There are about five hundred nations of indigenous people in North America, each representing a unique set of healing practices and knowledge. Nevertheless, there are still certain widely-held, general principles and beliefs among the many Native American tribes, about the nature of disease-producing behavior, healthy living and the spiritual values that reinstate balance and good health. These principles and beliefs are common among all the Native American tribes; albeit that the methods and techniques of diagnosis and of treatment vary among the tribes. But altogether, and as a unified and independent body of knowledge, the healing traditions of Native Americans have been practiced in North America since at least twelve thousand years ago and perhaps as early as forty thousand years ago.

Many practices and traditions of Native American healing have been kept hidden and undocumented. Instead the traditions have been passed down by oral tradition from elders to the youths, from the healers to their apprentices and from the guardian spirits to their vessels through visions and initiation. This method of passing down Native

American healing knowledge is deliberately methodical and slow. This is because the aim was to avoid transmitting healing knowledge too quickly, too willingly or too casually, as doing so would diminish the spiritual power of the herbs, remedies and medicines involved.

In any event, in contemporary times, many Native American healers and others with healing knowledge have begun to recognize the need to memorialize and document Native American healing practices and knowledge as a surer and safer way of ensuring that such important practices and knowledge are properly collected, verified and transferred to future generations.

In addition, many Native American healers and others with relevant knowledge have begun to see the virtue in sharing their special healing knowledge and values with the world as a special and invaluable Native American contribution to the welfare of the peoples of the world.

Native American medicine is immersed in a spiritual context, based on a spiritual conception of the world and life. In this world view, to be healthy, a person must be committed to a life of beauty, balance and harmony in all of the internal and the external. Generosity, gratitude, goodwill and respect are particularly regarded to be vital for a healthy life. Health is conceived as a state of balance and wholeness in the mind, spirit and body, where the balance produces wholeness and health. The balance is holistic, existing in the life energy in the body, in the exhibition of reasonable, just and ethical behavior, in the harmonious relations with self, family, community, nature, the environment and the world, physically, emotionally and spiritually. Thus a healthy person in the context of Native American medicine is a person who is, internally and externally, living in balance and harmony with all, under the guidance of the Great Spirit.

Also, in Native American medicine diseases may be thought to have either internal or external causes or in some cases, both. Among the internal causes of disease, negative thinking has been particularly identified as the most critical. Negative thinking includes negative self-talk, self-shame, self-blame, low self-esteem, depression, despair, hopelessness, greed, jealousy, envy, worry, anger, jealousy and selfishness, etc.

Some of the external causes of disease include germs, certain people, certain spirits, environmental poisons (such as air, water, soil pollution, drug abuse, food poisonings, environmental degradations), emotional, physical and spiritual trauma (leading to loss of a person's soul or spiritual power and emotional/mental problems), etc.

Germs are viewed not as mere microbes, but as active and reactive spirits that can infiltrate into a person and cause disease when certain conditions are present (such as when the person has allowed imbalance and dysfunction into their life or when the person has allowed their constitution to be persistently weak or when the person habitually engages in negative thinking or when the person has allowed pressure and stress to get the best of them.

Indeed, Native American medicine can physically, emotionally, and spiritually benefit anyone who sincerely wishes to live in wholeness and in healthier balance with nature, the environment and all forms of life. Indeed, Native American medicine can benefit and heal you.

Here are some basic guiding principles to the Native American healing process and concept of good health and wellness. And anyone who wishes to receive benefit and healing from the Native American healing process would do well to pay attention to these principles. And remember that the overarching aim of these guiding principles is to promote balance, harmony, wholeness, good medicine and maximum healing efficacy. Here are the principles:

1. Always acknowledge and show appreciation to God and for all the interconnectedness and relatedness of everything within and around you.

2. There is a purpose for everything and a thing (or means) for every purpose. Nothing goes for nothing. And everything is interconnected. (Basically, this explains why, to the Native American, healing goes way beyond the healing herb to include balance and harmony in many other aspects of our existence. Disease and illness are connected to imbalance and disharmony in some aspect of our existence).

3. Be charitable and give cheerfully to others when your needs and your family's needs have been met. (Basically we are all connected, so be concerned for the welfare of others and assist people when you can. And, of course, God loves a cheerful giver).

4. Pursue balance and harmony in everything. Practice, patience, silence, equanimity, self-control, self-respect, and fortitude. (Basically, always check your appetite for everything for excesses and govern yourself accordingly. Always respect yourself).

5. Practice the exchange of fair value. Give something back for everything you receive. Always seek permission, first and acknowledge and appreciate every living thing. (Basically, everything has an intrinsic value. Acknowledge and appreciate that value. And since nothing goes for nothing always exchange/pay fair value for whatever you take).

6. Respect people. Do not stare at people. Not staring at elders, community leaders and teachers is a sign of respect. (the actual meaning of this is to underscore the importance of respect in the scheme of required balance and harmony. Basically you should respect your parents, elders, leaders, bosses, experts, consultants, teachers and all those in position of authority over you).

7. Care for the earth as you would your mother. Protect, honor, revere, respect and give to the earth. She is your mother. (Basically, be environmentally conscious and endeavor to leave the environment in a better condition than you met it).

8.Listen to guidance. Listen to the guidance from your heart, your intuition, your subconscious and your spirit. And listen to wise guidance from others, including wise guidance from wise elders, wise mentors and wise friends. (Basically, do not face life's problems alone. Understand the great importance of relationships and social networks to your good health and wellbeing. And always look deep within yourself, as the solution to your problems may already be residing within you).

Furthermore, here are some of the discernible aspects of the Native American approach to healing, good health and wellness:

Healing and wellness are holistic

The Native American approach to healing and wellness is holistic. That is, they believe that healing and wellness involve not only the disease and the healing herb, but also the mind and the spirit of the patient and the energy in the community and in the environment. In short, you need to approach the Native American healing process, not with a mere transactional mindset, but with positive energy and a holistic mindset that accepts the connection of the disease, to the healing herb, to the patient, to the patient's mind, spirit and energy, to the energy of the community and to the energy in the environment. Everything is interconnected.

Healing and wellness are herbalistic

Native Americans believed in a herbalistic approach to healing and wellness. They used the herbs and medicinal plants in their environment not only for healing but also to balance their connection to their spirituality and overall wellbeing. Native Americans used herbs and medicinal plants for almost everything ranging from the prevention and curing of diseases, treatment of injuries and trauma, and as food and food flavorings. Native Americans believe in the efficacy of herbal remedies and used herbal remedies (before modern medicine) to heal wounds, treat illnesses and remain balanced and healthy.

Cleanliness is connected to good health and dirtiness is connected to disease

Native Americans understand that diseases thrive in filthy surroundings. Indeed, almost all of humanity's major plagues (e.g. small pox, influenza and many other communicable diseases) flourished and killed many people because of poor personal and public hygiene. So the Native American approach to healing includes an understanding of the connection between dirtiness and disease and between cleanliness and good health. Native Americans, therefore, aspire to high personal hygiene standards. The lesson here is that as you approach the Native American healing process, you should understand the exalted position of cleanliness and high personal hygiene standards in that healing process. And, of course, you need to continue to maintain such standards for a faster healing.

Healing and wellness are naturalistic and safe, yet effective

Native Americans believe in the sufficiency of nature. They believe that the environment contains all that they need to thrive. So they have a naturalistic (and minimalist) approach to everything, including healing. And this was very effective, because when the first settlers met Native Americans they observed that the Native Americans were successfully treating (with herbal remedies), many of the illnesses that were prevalent among their population. This Native American naturalistic, herbalistic, minimalist approach to healing has now become ever more important considering the issue of the side effects that come with modern pharmaceuticals. The bottom line here is that the Native American healing process is naturalistic. It uses ingredients straight from nature with little or no modification. This is a big advantage to you because it will enable you to be less worried about side effects and drug interactions, etc. But remember that natural does not always mean safe (particularly with regard to dosing). So ingesting the correct dose of even natural products is very important.

The body is sacred and food is medicine

Native Americans consider the body to be sacred and judge that only the healthiest, the most positive and the most spiritually agreeable foods should be introduced into the body. Native Americans also think of food as medicine and as an important aspect of the healing process. As a result, traditional Native American diet does not feature much processed foods or refined sugars. Instead it solely features whole foods, including vegetables, fruits, herbs, roots, nuts, seeds and lean meats. In addition, Native Americans typically, aspired to moderation even with eating, eschewing gluttony and greed.

As you learn more about Native American herbs, medicinal plants, herbal remedies and cures, remember the guiding principles and approaches listed above and endeavor to inculcate them in your life. They are all part of the Native American healing process and not only will they heal you, they will also hasten your healing, make your life more balanced and more harmonious and make you a happier, healthier person.

Now let's dive into the herbs and medicinal plants that constitute the bulk of Native American herbology.

CHAPTER 2: NATIVE AMERICAN HERBS AND MEDICINAL PLANTS AND THEIR SPECIFIC USES IN THE HEALING OF DIFFERENT DISEASES AND CONDITIONS

Abcess Root (*Polemonium reptans*). This plant is also called American Greek valerian, sweatroot, spreading Jacob's ladder, false Jacob's ladder, blue bells, creeping Jacob's ladder or stairway to heaven. The Meskwaki Native American tribe used this plant as a cathartic and a Diuretic. They made a compound containing the root of this plant and used it as a strong physic and a urinary aid. An infusion or a tincture (in alcohol) of the dried roots of this plant has also been used internally to treat tuberculosis, colds, coughs, fever, laryngitis, bronchitis, poisonous bites, skin conditions and inflammatory diseases. A decoction made from the entire plant has also been used as a hair rinse. To make an abcess root tea/ infusion, steep 1 teaspoon of dried root of abcess root in 1 cup of water for about 10 minutes and enjoy. It's good for colds, coughs, and congestions. This plant can be found in eastern North America (from Minnesota, to Kansas to New York to Georgia).

Agrimony (*Agrimonia eupatoria*). CAUTION. Do not consume if pregnant or breast feeding. Also do not consume in large quantities as doing so could cause constipation and other digestive issues due to the presence of tannins in this plant. The seed of this pant is edible but is mostly considered a famine food. The dried or fresh flowers, leaves and stem have been used to make tea. Agrimony aids digestion and is effective against diarrhea. An infusion of this plan taken internally has also been used to treat jaundice and other liver problems and as a gargle to treat sore throats and inflammation of the mouth, pharynx and skin. A decoction is applied externally to treat skin problems, wounds and hemorrhoids, etc.

Akebia (*Akebia quinata*). This plant is also called fiveleaf akebia or chocolate vine. The fruit, leaves and shoots are edible. The fruits and the young shoots can be eaten raw. The young shoots can be pickled or added into salads and eaten. The leaves have been consumed as a tea substitute. Akebia is antibacterial and antifungal and is taken to treat urinary tract infections. It is also taken to improve lactation, to stimulate menstruation, to treat edema and rheumatism and as a remedy for cancer (particularly lung cancer). Also, the root is ingested to ease fevers. This plant is invasive to North America and can be found in the eastern North America (Georgia, Massachusetts to Michigan).

Alabama serviceberry (*Amelanchier arborea*). This plant is also called by the following names: juneberry, downy serviceberry or common serviceberry. It can be found in eastern North America (New Brunswick to Florida and Minnesota to Texas). The fruit of this plant is edible and can be eaten cooked or raw. The Cherokee ate the fruit/berries of this plant for food. The Blackfoot also ate the dried berries as food (especially together with meat). The Blackfoot also used the berries in soups and stews. The Cherokee used this plant medicinally in different ways. They used this plant as an anthelmintic by ingesting a compound infusion of the plant to eliminate worms. They also took a compound infusion internally to treat diarrhea and they took the compound infusion as a spring tonic. The Iroquois used this plant as a venereal aid (particularly to treat gonorrhea). They also used the plant as a gynecological aid, by giving the fruits (or an infusion made from the small branches of this plant) to new mothers (right after giving birth) as a remedy for hemorrhages and the after-pains of childbirth. The Iroquois have also used the fruits of this plant as a blood medicine.

Alaska bog willow (*Salix fuscescens*). This flowering shrub is native to northern, North America and can be found in Alaska (except the southeastern coast and in the Aleutian Islands) and in northern Canada). Alaska bog willow (like all willows) contain salacin, which is directly linked to aspirin. Generally, Native Americans used this plant to treat diarrhea, bee stings, toothaches and stomach aches. The Eskimo used the Alaska bog willow as an eye medicine. Cotton soaked in an infusion of the plant was placed on the inner corner of the eyes to treat sore, watery eyes. The Eskimo also chewed the leaves of this plant to treat mouth sores.

Alfalfa (*Medicago sativa*). CAUTION.Avoid Alfalfa if you have an auto-immune condition.

Nevertheless, alfalfa has been utilized in herbal medicine for centuries. Indeed, it is an old Native American medicine for blood clotting and treating jaundice. It is currently also used for treating several other health issues including: muscle problems, arthritis, kidney and bladder problems, reduction of blood sugar levels, menopause problems, eliminating toxins increasing energy and bone issues.

Allspice (*Calycanthus floridus*). This plant is also known as Carolina allspice, sweetshrub, eastern sweetshrub or strawberry bush. The Cherokee have used the ooze that comes out of the bark of this plant to treat pediatric sores. They have also used an infusion of the plant to treat hives. They have used the roots of this plant as a powerful emetic and to treat bladder and urinary problems. A cold infusion made from the bark has also been used by the Cherokee as eye drops to prevent loss of eyesight. This plant can be found in south-eastern North America (from Virginia to Florida to West Virginia and Alberta).

American Aspen (*Populus tremuloides*). CAUTION. Possible toxic effects due to the presence of salicylates in this plant (e.g. heartburn, tinnitus). Avoid if you suffer from ulcers, stomach or peptic ulcers. Handle or use only under the supervision of a licensed doctor. American aspen has been used by Native Americans for the treatment of wounds, skin complaints and respiratory disorders. American Aspen is used internally for the treatment of arthritis, rheumatism, lower back pains, liver and digestive disorders, gout, urinary complaints, anorexia, debility, to reduce fevers and to relieve menstrual cramps and pains. Used externally, the bark is effective against hemorrhoids, chilblains, sprains and infected wounds. An infusion of the inner bark is used as an appetite stimulant and a cough remedy. It is also used in the treatment of urinary ailments, venereal disease, worms, stomach pains, colds and fevers.

American Mistletoe (*Phoradendron leucarpum*). Native Americans have used this herb for lung problems, blood pressure, headache, epilepsy, abortions and as a contraceptive. The Cherokee Indians made a tea of this herb and used it to bathe the head for headaches. The Creek Indians made a decoction of this herb that was helpful for lung troubles, including tuberculosis. The Mendocino Indians also used the root of this plant to prevent conception and to induce abortions. Other uses included rubbing the body with a decoction of the leaves for painful joints and limbs and chewing on the root for toothaches. American Mistletoe was also used by some Native American tribes in religious ceremonies. This plant is considered poisonous and should be handled with caution.

American Turkey Oak (*Quercus laevis*). This tree is also called turkey oak. This tree can be found in south-eastern North America (from Louisiana, Florida to Virginia). The seeds of this tree are edible and eaten cooked. The seeds can be dried, ground, powdered and mixed with flours to make bread or used as thickening for stews. This tree produces galls that are very astringent and they have been used to treat chronic diarrhea, hemorrhages and dysentery. This tree is also used to treat bladder and kidney problems (including Bright's disease), diarrhea, viral infections, menstrual issues, sprains, swellings, sores and as a booster for other therapies.

Antelope Sage (*Eriogonum Jamesii*). The Navajo Native American tribe have used Antelope Sage as a contraceptive. One cup of the roots-decoction was also taken internally by the women during menstruation. A decoction of the whole plant has also been used to relieve the pain of childbirth and the root has been masticated or used in teas as a cardiac medicine, for depression and for stomach aches. A wash was also made with this herb to treat sore eyes.

Barren Strawberry (*Waldsteinia fragarioides*). A compound decoction of Barren Strawberry is taken for blood issues. The poultice of the smashed plant is also applied to snakebites. This plant is native to eastern North America and can be found from Minnesota, Quebec, Ontario and Maine south to Pennsylvania and Indiana and further on south to the mountains of North Carolina.

Bergamot (*Monarda* fistulosa). Native American tribes have used this plant to remedy various medical complaints including digestive-system disorders. An infusion is used internally to treat gastric disorders, colds, catarrh, aching kidneys, headaches, fevers and sore throat. Externally, a poultice of this plant is used to treat cuts, abrasions, boils and skin eruptions, etc. A wash made from this plant is also used for sore eyes. The leaves can be used dried or fresh. Essential oil from this plant has also been inhaled to treat bronchial problems and to flush out gas from the digestive tract. This plant can be found around North-eastern North America (from Quebec to Minnesota, south to Texas).

Black chokecherry (*Prunus virginiana*). This plant is also called chokecherry or western chokecherry. CAUTION: The seed of this plant contains hydrogen cyanide, a poison. If only a small quantity of hydrogen cyanide is ingested, it can stimulate respiration and improve digestion. But when ingested in excess, it can cause respiratory distress and possibly, death. The fruit and the seed of this plant are edible. The fruit and the seed can both be eaten either cooked or raw. But do not eat the seed at all if it is too bitter as the bitterness indicates the presence of high levels of hydrogen cyanide, a poison, in the seed which can be fatal if eaten in excess. See notes above under "caution". Also, a tea can be made out of the twigs and the bark.

Nevertheless, Native Americans used this plant to treat a variety of complaints including: using it to treat issues of the respiratory system; using it to treat wounds (inner bark; ingesting it to treat laryngitis and stomach complaints (inner bark decoction); using it to wash old sores, burns and ulcers. (inner bark infusion); taking the fruit juice to treat sore throat; powdering the fruit and taking it as a treatment for bloody bowel excretions, diarrhea and as an appetite stimulant; using the bark to treat wounds, sores, cough, cold, sore throat, diarrhea, tuberculosis, scrofula, hemoptysis, piles and stomach cramps; steaming and inhaling the bark to treat snow blindness and smoking the bark to treat head cold and headache.

Black Cohosh (*Cimicifuga Racemosa*). Native Americans, including the Winnebago, Dakota, and the Oklahoma Delaware have used the root of the plant in decoctions and teas to treat gynecological issues, kidney problems, depression, cough, sore throats and headache. Even today, it continues to be used for gynecological problems, including menopause and pre-menstrual tension, as well as respiratory ailments, nervous conditions, arthritis, tinnitus, sciatica, aches and colds.

Black Gum (*Nyssa Sylvatica*). This tree is also commonly known as tupelo or pepperide. Its bark, fruit and roots have been used by Native Americans in decoctions to treat eye problems, induce vomiting and eliminate worms in children and as a bath. The Cherokee Native American tribe have used a mild tea made from small twigs and the bark from this tree to ease chest pain.

Black haw (*Viburnum prunifolium*). CAUTION: Overdose symptoms include: dizziness, nausea, visual disturbances, reduced pulse rate, increased perspiration and fits (seizures). Rare allergic reactions. Avoid this herb if pregnant due to the herb's effects on the uterus. Nonetheless, an infusion made from the bark of this plant has been used as a wash for sore tongues. An infusion of the root bark is used as a tonic and a diaphoretic. An infusion taken internally is considered effective as prevention against persistent spasms and a compound infusion is also taken internally to treat smallpox, fever and ague. This plant can be found in Eastern North America (from Connecticut to Florida, west to and Kansas).

Black Horehound (*Ballota* nigra). This herb has been used for the treatment of menopause problems, menstrual disorders, bronchial complaints, respiratory issues, nervous dyspepsia, depression, convulsions, travelling sickness, arthritis, morning sickness in pregnancy, gout, and as an antiemetic. This herb should not be put in storage for more than one year. The fresh herb is sometimes used to prepare a syrup.

Blue Cohosh (*Caulophyllum* Thalictroides). Native Americans have long used the root in tonics and teas to treat uterine problems, female reproductive issues, to induce labor, to relieve the pains of childbirth and to treat rheumatism, colic, dropsy, hiccough, cramps and epilepsy. Several Native American tribes have also used Blue Cohosh together with other herbs and remedies for contraceptive and abortive purposes.

California Broomrape (*Orobanche californica*). A decoction of this herb has been used to treat pneumonia, colds and pulmonary complaints. This plant can be found in the South-western North America (from British Columbia and Idaho, through California and Nevada, to Baja California).

California False Hellebore (*Veratrum californicum*). CAUTION: This plant is highly poisonous. Handle or use only under the supervision of a licensed doctor. Native American

Indian tribes have applied this plant externally to treat wounds. It has also been used as a contraceptive. A decoction of this plant has also been used as treatment for venereal disease. The roots have been shredded, then chewed and the juice ingested as a treatment for colds. The roots have been dried and ground up and applied as dressing for sores and bruises. A poultice of the pulverized raw root has been applied as treatment for sores, boils, cuts, burns, swellings and rheumatism. A decoction of the root has been ingested (by both women and men) for a contraceptive. But beware, one teaspoon of this root decoction, if taken 3 times per day for 3 weeks, is believed to cause permanent sterility in women!

Caper (*Capparis spinose*). The root-bark of this plant is used internally for the treatment of gastrointestinal infections, gout, rheumatism and diarrhea. The unopened flower buds of this plant are used internally in the treatment of coughs and as a laxative. The flower buds are also used externally to treat eye infections. And the buds may be preventive of the formation of cataracts. The stem bark will increase the appetite, if taken before meals. The plant is used externally to treat capillary weakness and easy bruising and other skin conditions. A decoction of the plant has been used as treatment for vaginal thrush, while a poultice of the leaves has been used to treat gout.

Carolina vetch (*Vicia caroliniana*). This plant is used to treat back pains, local pains, muscle cramps, twitching and to strengthen the muscles. It is also rubbed on the stomach for stomach cramps. It is also rubbed on for rheumatism. It is also used internally with rabbit tobacco, sweet everlasting for rheumatism. An infusion of this plant is effective against muscle pain. It is also used an emetic.

Cheeseweed (*Malva parviflora*). This plant has been used as a poultice on boils, swellings and sores. The seeds are used in the treatment of bladder ulcers and coughs. And a decoction of the leaves or roots has been used as a hair rinse to soften the hair and to remove dandruff from the hair.

Chicory (*Cichorium intybus*). CAUTION: Excessive and/or prolonged use of this plant may impair the retina and cause sensitization. Nevertheless, an infusion of the root of this plant has been used as a nerve tonic. A decoction of the roots has also been used as a wash (also applied as a poultice) on fever sores and chancres. This plant is not native to the Americas and was introduced by the settlers.

Clasping bellwort (*Triodanis perfoliata*). An infusion of the roots of this plant has been taken internally, also used as a bath for dyspepsia. The root has also been used in a liquid compound for dyspepsia from overeating. This plant is native to North and South America (from Canada to Argentina).

Crested iris (*Iris cristata*). A decoction of the pulverized root is used as salve for ulcers. A decoction of the root has also been used to treat yellow urine. The root is also used as a poultice and in various other formulations to apply to skin ulcers.

And an infusion of the plant is used to treat liver complaints.

Crinkleroot, Common toothworth (*Cardamine diphylla*). An infusion of the whole plant is taken for breast health. The Iroquois Native American tribe also chewed the raw root and swallowed the juice to treat stomach gas. A poultice of the roots has been applied to swellings for pain and inflammation relief. A cold infusion of the plant has been taken internally for fever, heart palpitations and chest pain. Also an infusion of the plant taken at the beginning of tuberculosis has been found to be helpful.

Damiana (*Turnera Diffusa*). This herb is claimed to stimulate the libido and has been used as an aphrodisiac. It has also been used to improve digestion, increase energy, treat impotence, depression, nervousness, anxiety, asthma, constipation and menstrual problems.

Day Flower (*Commelina communis*). This plant has been prepared as a gargle and used to treat tonsillitis and sore throat. A decoction of the dried plant is used to treat diarrhea, bleeding and fever etc. Extracts of this plant has shown antibacterial activity.

Dogwood (*Cornus Florida*). The berries, inner bark and twigs from this tree have long been used in Native American herbology. Dogwood was used internally to treat pneumonia, fever, malaria, diarrhea and colds, as well as to improve appetite and digestion. A poultice of the plant was used to treat sores and ulcers. The Iroquois Native American tribe have used a tonic prepared from the twigs of this plant to treat gonorrhea. The Cherokee Native American tribe chewed the bark of the tree for headache relief. They also used a decoction of the bark to treat childhood afflictions (such as measles, worms and diarrhea). The Cherokee also made poultices of this plant, which were used for treating wounds and other skin disorders.

Dropwort (*Filipendula vulgaris*). This plant's anti-inflammatory, antioxidant, antipyretic, anti-rheumatic, anti-ulcer and gastro-protective properties have been confirmed by scientific studies. The root of this plant is used in the treatment of bladder and kidney stones, intestinal worms, genital discharges and epilepsy. Suitable habitats for this plant include forest edges, glades, meadows, forest-steppe zones and meadow steppes in the forest.

Dwarf cinquefoil (*Potentilla Canadensis*). This plant is also called running five fingers or Canadian dwarf cinquefoil. It is a perennial, a wild flower, a weed, an herb and a native plant of Northern America. The Iroquois Native American tribe have used an infusion of the roots of this plant as an antidiarrheal. This plant can be found in North America (around Connecticut, Maine, Massachusetts, New Hampshire, Rhode Island and Vermont).

Elder (*Sambucus*). There are several species in the Sambucus family. But the commonly used specie among the Native American tribes is the Black Elderberry (*Sambucus Canadensis*). CAUTION:

This plant is poisonous, particularly the stems and leaves. Its fruit has caused stomach discomfort in some people. The unripe fruit contains toxins. So handle and use this plant with care and only under the supervision of a licensed doctor. Nevertheless, the dried flowers and berries have been used in tonics and teas to treat flu and constipation. The Cherokee and the Delaware Native American tribes made a tea from the dried flowers of this plant to sweat out toxins. The Seminole and the Creek Native American tribes pounded the root of this plant to utilize as a topical treatment for swelling. But remember that some caution should be exercised if any part of this plant is being used fresh. It can cause poisoning.

Eulalia (*Miscanthus sinensis*). The juice of young stems is used to diffuse and dispel poisons, blood clots, extravagated blood and to relieve inflammation.

Evergreen Huckleberry (*Vaccinium ovatum*). A decoction of the leaves of this plant has been used in the treatment of diabetes. An infusion of the leaves and sugar have also been given to a mother after childbirth to help restore her strength.

Everlasting Flower (*Helichrysum arenarium*). An infusion of this plant is used as a diuretic and in treating cystitis, rheumatism and gall bladder disorders, etc. A homeopathic remedy, made from the flowering plant, is also used to treat lumbago and gall bladder disorders.

Fendler's Bladderpod (*Lesquerella fendleri*). This plant has been used by the Hopi Native American tribe as a gynecological aid after childbirth and to induce vomiting. The Navajo and the Kayenta Native American tribes also used a poultice of the roots of this plant to treat sore eyes. The Navajo also used the plant as a snuff to clear nasal passages and as a poultice of pulverized leaves to treat spider bites and toothaches.

Feverfew (*Tanacetum Parthenium*). CAUTION: Feverfew may interfere with medications and should not be used without first consulting your doctor. Prolonged use followed by a sudden cessation may induce a withdrawal condition including headaches and joint and muscle pains. Some people are allergic to feverfew. And feverfew should be avoided by women during pregnancy. Nevertheless, feverfew has long been used to reduce fever and to treat migraines, headaches, digestive problems and arthritis. It has also been used to treat labor difficulties, menstrual irregularities, stomach aches, skin conditions, and asthma.

Feverwort (*Triosteum Perfoliatum*). This plant has been used to treat nausea, diarrhea, back pain, flu, joint stiffness, nervous symptoms, welts, itching and pleurisy. The Cherokee also ingested a decoction of the herb to cure fever.

Few-seeded sedge (Carex oligosperma). A compound decoction of the plant is used as an emetic (an agent that induces vomiting).

Frost Grape (*Vitis vulpine*). The leaves of this plant have been used to treat liver disorders. The wilted leaves have been applied as a poultice to the breasts to relieve soreness after birth. An infusion of the bark has been used to treat urinary problems. And an infusion of the roots has also been taken to treat diabetes and rheumatism.

Galbanum (*Ferula gummosa*). The roots of this plant (including the whole plant) contain the gum resin, "galbanum". Internally, it is used to treat asthma, chronic bronchitis, pulmonary issues and other chest complaints. It also acts as a digestive stimulant and relieves flatulence, colic and griping pains. Externally it is used as a plaster for ulcers, wounds, boils, inflammatory swellings and various skin complaints.

Garden Pea (*Pisum sativum*). This plant has been used as a contraceptive. The seed-oil, ingested by women, once a month, has been used as a contraceptive to prevent pregnancy. It works by hampering the workings of progesterone. In trials, the seed-oil reduced pregnancy rate in women by 60% in a 2-year period and reduced male sperm count by 50% in the same 2-year period. The seed-oil also inhibits endometrial development. Furthermore, a poultice (of the dried and powdered seed of this plant) has been used on the skin to treat acne and other skin problems.

Giant buttercup (*Ranunculus acris*). This plant is also called tall buttercup, meadow buttercup and Showy buttercup. CAUTION: Every part of this plant is poisonous, although the toxins can be deteriorated and destroyed by drying or heating. Contact with the plant juice may trigger a blistering of the skin. Indeed, the entire plant is very acrid and can burn the mucous membranes including the mouth. Nevertheless, this plant has been used as a poultice (rubbed on) to treat chest pain, abscess, boils, rheumatism and cold. The flowers and the leaves have been mashed and inhaled to treat headaches. An infusion made from the roots is taken for diarrhea. Its sap has been utilized as a sedative and for wart removal.

Goat's Beard (*Tragopogon* pratensis). Goat's beard is considered effective for the treatment of liver and gallbladder issues. It is high in inulin and as such is good food for diabetics (inulin does not increase blood sugar levels). Goat's Beard also appears to stimulate digestion and the appetite and it may also be effective as a detoxifying agent. A decoction of the root is ingested to treat heartburn, loss of appetite and disorders of the breast or liver and a syrup made from the root provides relief in cases of bronchitis and persistent coughs. Fresh juice made from the young plant is used to dissolve bile and to relieve the stomach.

Goldenrod, wrinkle leaf (*Solidago rugose*). The whole plant is used as liver medicine and for biliousness. A decoction of its leaves and flowers is used for weakness, dizziness or sunstroke.

Goldenseal (*Hydrastis Canadensis*). This plant is used in cancer treatment.

Gray hydrangea, ashy (*Hydrangea cinerea*). An infusion of the bark scrapings is ingested for vomiting bile. An infusion of the roots is also ingested as an emetic and a cathartic by women during mensuration.

Great Burdock (*Arctium lappa*). This plant is also known as gobo. CAUTION: Avoid burdock if pregnant or breastfeeding. Also, the tiny hairs on the seeds are toxic and can be inhaled if one is not careful. Inhaling the hairs can trigger allergic reactions. Burdock is naturalized in North America. The leaves, seed, root and stem of this plant are all edible. The root can be eaten cooked or raw and can be dried and stored for later use. The young leaves and young branches and stalks can also be eaten cooked or raw. The seeds can also be sprouted and eaten somewhat like bean-sprouts.

Burdock is one of the best blood-purifying and detoxifying herbs. The dried root of the young plant, the fruits and the leaves are used in herbal medicine and are very effective against ailments that have to do with excess toxins in the system. The root is particularly effective at helping to remove heavy metals from the system. Burdock is also included in the Essiac formula which is popularly used to treat cancer. Burdock is carminative, antibacterial and antifungal and also very effective for various skin problems, bruises and burns. It is also used to treat eczema, herpes, impetigo, acne, bites, boils and ringworm, etc. The seed extracts also decrease blood sugar levels. Burdock can be made into an infusion and ingested or externally used as a wash. A poultice can also be made of the pulverized seed and applied to bruises. A poultice of the leaves can also be applied to treat ulcers, sores and burns.

In Native American herbology, the Cherokee used the plant to treat rheumatism, gravel and scurvy. They also took an infusion of the seeds or root to purify the blood and to treat venereal disease. The Malecite combined smashed burdock roots and gilead buds to treat sores. The Malecite also used an infusion of the buds to treat chancre. A decoction of the plant has been used by the Otos to treat pleurisy and Meskwaki women have used the burdock root to ease labor. The Potawatomis made a tea of burdock root and drank it as a blood purifier and tonic. The Flambeau Ojibwa used burdock root along with other herbs to treat stomach pain and they also drank it as a tonic. The Menominee applied a poultice of boiled burdock leaves to treat scrofulous sores on the neck. They also used it as a remedy for tuberculosis. The Micmac used burdock roots and buds to treat sores and chancre. And the Ojibwa used burdock roots as a blood medicine. Burdock is also helpful with cancer and Alzheimer's disease.

Greater celandine, nipplewort, swallowwort (*Chelidonium majus*). CAUTION: Greater celandine is a toxic plant. It is generally not recommended for internal use unless under strict supervision of a licensed doctor. Nevertheless, traditionally Greater celandine has been used to treat a number of digestive issues including constipation, irritable bowel syndrome, gastroenteritis and stomach upset. It is also used to boost the appetite. By the way, modern research findings now suggest that the plant has anti-cancer potentials as it destroys cancer cells through apoptosis.

Hard Stem Bulrush (*Scirpus acutus*). The root of this perennial can be eaten cooked or raw, often it is ground, powdered and mixed with cereal to make bread. The root can also be boiled into a syrup. The pollen is also edible and is mixed with flour to make cake, bread, etc. The young shoots and the inner parts of the stems are also edible, raw or cooked.

A poultice of this plant has been used to stop wound bleeding. The roots have also been chewed to prevent thirst. This plant can be found in North America (Canada and southwards).

Honeysuckle (*Lonicera periclymenum*). Honeysuckle has been used as a laxative and as an expectorant. A syrup produced from the flowers has been used to treat respiratory diseases and a decoction of the leaves has been used to treat diseases of the spleen and liver. It is also used in gargles and as a mouthwash for ulcers.

Hooked agrimony, common agrimony (*Agrimonia gryposepala*). This plant is used to treat fever. The Iroquois also used a drink made from the roots of this plant to treat diarrhea.

Horehound (*Marrubium Vulgare*). CAUTION: People with peptic ulcer issues or gastritis should use this plant only under the supervision of a licensed doctor. Avoid any pediatric use of the seeds, as there has been at least one instance where the seeds have poisoned children who ate them. Nevertheless, this plant has been long used to treat several ailments including digestive disorders. It has also been used as an expectorant and as a cough suppressant. Other uses include for the treatment of gastric problems, constipation, flatulence, indigestion, painful menstruation, asthma, bronchitis, colds, cough, nausea, whooping cough and tuberculosis. Horehound is also used as an appetite stimulant and as a sedative. Externally, horehound has been used to treat sores, abrasions and skin disorders and as a cleansing agent for wounds.

Horsemint (*Mentha Longifolia*). CAUTION: Horsemint should not be used by pregnant women. Nevertheless, this plant has been used for its effect on digestion and for its antiseptic properties. The flowering stems and leaves have been used in tonics and teas to treat headaches, fever, chills, inflammation, menstrual disorders, colic, cough, flatulence, congestion, urinary tract infections and cold. Horsemint has also been used to induce labor and as a stimulant. It has been used externally on sores, swellings and minor wounds. The stems and leaves of this plant were combined in boiling water and the vapors were inhaled to alleviate nasal and bronchial congestion. Many Native American tribes have used this plant to treat fever, inflammation and chills. The Catawba drank an infusion of the leaves to treat back pain.

Hound's tongue (*Cynoglossum officinale*). CAUTION: While hound's tongue has been used in the treatment of cancer, it can also be carcinogenic if taken internally, in large doses. Nevertheless, hound's tongue contains allantoin, a highly effective agent that speeds up the healing process in the body. This plant also has a wide antitumor reputation for cancers of various types. It has also been used as a pain reliever. Hound's tongue has also been used internally in the treatment of coughs and diarrhea. It has also been used as a poultice on piles, wounds, minor injuries, bites and ulcers. A homeopathic remedy made from the roots of this plant has also been used and is very effective in the treatment of insomnia.

Ice plant (*Mesembryanthemum crystallinum*). This plant has been used to treat inflammations of the genito-urinary and pulmonary mucous membranes. The leaves have also been used in the treatment of dysentery, ascites and diseases of the kidney and liver.

Indian hemp (*Apocynum Cannabinum*). This herb is a specie of marijuana. It is native all over much of North America. It is a toxic plant and if consumed can trigger cardiac arrest. But Indian hemp has been used by Native Americans in the preparation of herbal remedies. Its boiled roots were made into teas and decoctions to treat syphilis, asthma, rheumatism, fever, dysentery and intestinal worms. The Prairie Potawatomi Indians also used this herb to treat dropsy and as a heart medicine.

Indian Paintbrush (*Castilleja*). The Chippewa Indians have used Indian Paintbrush to treat rheumatism. They have also used it in a bath rinse to make their hair glossy. The Nevada Indians used the plant to enhance the immune system and for the treatment of sexually-transmitted diseases. Hopi Indian women drank a tea made from the whole plant to halt or quicken menstrual flow.

Indigo weed, rattlebush (*Baptisia australis*). CAUTION: Potential toxicity of this plant has been related. So, handle and use with care and only under the supervision of a licensed doctor. The roots of this plant have been used in an herbal tea as a purgative or to treat nausea and toothaches. The plant is under investigation for potential immunostimulating properties. This plant can be found in Eastern and Central North America (from Pennsylvania to Georgia, west to Texas, Nebraska and Indiana).

Interrupted fern (*Osmunda claytoniana*). CAUTION: This plant may contain thiaminase (an enzyme that depletes vitamin B-complex). It may also contain carcinogens. Therefore, this plant should not be ingested in large quantities as it could be harmful. Nevertheless, this plant is used to treat venereal diseases and blood diseases. The Iroquois Indians have also used this plant as treatment for rickets and gonorrhea.

Ivy Gourd (*Coccinia grandis*). Juice made with the leaves and roots of this plant has been used to treat diabetes. The juice of the stem has also been dribbled into the eyes to remedy cataracts. The leaves have also been used as a poultice to treat skin eruptions. The plant is ingested to treat gonorrhea.

Japanese Chaff Flower (*Achyranthes japonica*). The root of this plant has been used to treat delayed menses. The root also contains analgesic, anti-allergic, anti-inflammatory, antispasmodic, diuretic, uterine stimulant and hypotensive properties.

Jerusalem artichoke (*Helianthus tuberosus*). This plant has been used as an aphrodisiac, diuretic, aperient, spermatogenetic, tonic and stomachic. Jerusalem artichoke is also a folk remedy for rheumatism and diabetes.

Jiaogulan (*Gynostemma Pentaphyllum*). This plant has cell-protective and anti-aging properties. It has been used to strengthen the immune system, lower high blood pressure and high cholesterol levels, improve the digestive and the reproductive systems, boost mental functions and liver functions and used to treat stress-related symptoms. This plant also inhibits the advancement of cancer.

Juniper (*Juniperus Communis*). CAUTION: consuming large doses of juniper can enflame the urinary tract. Also, pregnant women shouldn't use this plant as it has been known to cause miscarriages. Nevertheless, the small, round, blue-black berries that the female tree produces, may be consumed raw when properly ripe or made into a tea and consumed as treatment for rheumatic conditions, digestive disorders, high blood pressure, arthritis, gum disease, gout, bladder, kidney and urinary tract issues, diarrhea, dandruff and gonorrhea. Externally, juniper is applied in the form of a diluted oil on wounds and arthritic joints.

Kansas Hawthorn (*Crataegus coccinoides*). The flowers and fruits of this plant have a hypotensive effect. They also act as a heart tonic. They are especially indicated for the treatment of weak heart with high blood pressure. A prolonged use of the Kansas Hawthorn is usually required before it can become efficacious. It is normally used as either tincture or tea.

Katrafay (*Cedrelopsis grevei*). This plant is also called Kathrafay. The essential oil obtained from the bark of this tree has a wide range of medicinal applications. The bark extract has been shown to hold antibacterial and antifungal properties. Katrafay is also used to treat broken bones, toothache, rheumatism, arthritis, muscular pain and general body pain. It is also used as a vaginal wash, post-childbirth, because of its tonic effects.

Kendyr (*Apocynum pictum***).** The leaves yield up to 5% gum which is used for making a medicine used as a sedative and to treat hypertension.

Knawel (*Scleranthus annuus*). This plant has been used to treat "indecision", "uncertainty", "unbalance" and "hesitancy", where the patient is up and down in mood, experiencing extremes of joy/sadness, energy/apathy, optimism/pessimism, laughing, crying, etc. Knawel improves decisiveness and ability to make quick decisions and to act promptly when necessary.

Koa *(Acacia koa).* The bark was applied to abscesses, burst sores, ulcers, scars, sore tuberculosis adenitis, syphilis, leprosy, sore bruises, and broken bones.

Labrador Rose (*Rosa blanda*). A decoction of the fruit of this plant has been used to treat itching piles and other itches. The skin of the fruit has been used in the treatment of indigestion and stomach problems. The dried powdered flowers have been used to treat heartburn. An infusion of the root has been used as a wash to treat inflamed eyes. The infusion has also been used as an analgesic to treat lumbago and headaches. This plant is currently being investigated as a food that is capable of reducing the prevalence of cancer and as a way of halting or reversing the metastasis of cancers.

Lady Fern (*Athyrium filix-femina*). A tea of the boiled stems of this plant has been used to relieve labor pains. The fledgling, tender, unfurled fronds of this plant have also been eaten to treat internal ailments such as uterine cancer. A tea produced of the roots has been used to treat post-childbirth breast pains and general body pains and to stimulate milk flow in coagulated breasts. The dried powdered root has been applied on sores.

Lopseed (*Phryma leptostachya*). A tea made from the roots was gargled as a treatment for sore throats and was ingested to treat fevers, rheumatism, etc. A poultice made from the roots is applied to boils, carbuncles, sores and cancers.

Lime Berry (*Triphasia trifolia*). The leaves of this plant are applied to the body for the treatment of colic, skin diseases and diarrhea.

Madonna Lily (*Lilium candidum*). The plant is used mostly, externally. It is applied as a poultice on ulcers, tumors and external inflammations etc. The flowers are harvested when they have fully opened and are used while fresh to make ointments, juice or tinctures. The flower pollen has been used to treat epilepsy. The bulbs are harvested around August and can be used dried or fresh as medicines.

Malabar Gourd (*Cucurbita ficifolia*). This plant is anti-parasitic. The complete seed, together with the husk is ground into a fine flour, water is added and it is made into an emulsion and eaten. Thereafter a purgative is taken in order to expel worms and other parasites from the stomach. The plant is used as a remedy for eliminating internal parasites.

Mayapple (*Podophyllum Peltatum*). CAUTION: The ripened fruit of the mayapple is edible in moderate quantities, but can become poisonous when consumed in large amounts. Besides the ripened fruit which may be edible as explained above, all other parts of this plant are poisonous. And because of its toxicity, this herb should only be used by licensed professionals. Nevertheless, Native Americans have eaten the edible, ripened fruit of this plant cooked or raw. Although the remaining parts of the plant are toxic, Native Americans, nevertheless, knew how to use the roots of this plant to treat worms, liver issues and as a laxative. They also used the plant, externally, to treat warts, snakebite and some skin conditions. The ripened fruit of this plant is made into jellies, jams, pies and marmalades.

Mayflower (*Epigaea repens*). This plant is also called ground laurel or trailing arbutus. CAUTION: This plant contains arbutin which hydrolyzes to the toxin hydroquinone. Nevertheless, the flowers of the mayflower are edible and can be eaten raw. This plant has strong antiseptic properties and is particularly effective against urethritis, cystitis, bladder stones and prostatitis. An infusion of the leaves has been used to treat stomach aches, bladder and kidney disorders and blood/pus in the urine. An infusion is also used to treat kidney and chest complaints and pediatric diarrhea. A decoction (or compound infusion) of the leaves is also used to treat indigestion and to relieve labor pains in childbirth. A compound decoction of this pant is used to treat rheumatism. A decoction is also used for abdominal pain and to cause vomiting.

Maypops (*Passiflora incarnate*). CAUTION: Do not use this plant during pregnancy. Maypops is frequently used in the treatment of epilepsy, insomnia and hysteria etc. The stems and leaves are also used to treat women's complaints. The plant is also used in the treatment of nervous tension, insomnia, neuralgia, irritability, irritable bowel syndrome, vaginal discharges and pre-menstrual tension. A poultice of the roots is applied to earaches, cuts, boils and inflamed areas, etc.

Meadow buttercup (*Ranunculus acris*). CAUTION: All parts of this plant are poisonous (although the toxins can be destroyed by heat or by drying). The plant has a strong, acrid juice that can cause blistering to the skin. Indeed, the whole plant is extremely acrid and can cause intense pain and a burning sensation in the mouth and the mucous membranes etc. Nevertheless, a poultice of this plant is applied topically to the chest for colds and pains and to abscesses and boils. The leaves and the flowers of this plant have been pulverized and inhaled as treatment for headaches. The fresh leaves have also been pulverized, but applied topically to treat rheumatism. The sap of this plant has also been used to remove warts and as a sedative.

Meadow zizia (*Zizia aptera*). The Zizia species have potential medicinal value. Native Americans have used *Zizia* aurea roots made into tea to treat fevers. The plant is also used as an effective wound-healing agent.

Milkweed (*Asclepias Syriaca*). This herb has been used both as food and as medicine. CAUTION: This herb can be toxic if not prepared properly. Indeed, it may be toxic when taken internally, without sufficient preparation. Handle and use only under the supervision of a licensed doctor. The Meskwaki Indians and the Mohawk Indians used a decoction as a contraceptive; the Iroquois Indians and the Navajo Indians used it to prevent problems after childbirth. The Chippewa used it to produce postpartum milk flow. Other uses include, taken internally as treatment for female issues, stomach problems and chest discomfort. Or used externally to treat ringworm, warts and bee stings.

Narrowleaf cattail (*Typha angustifolia*). CAUTION: This plant should not be used while pregnant. Nevertheless, narrowleaf cattail is used internally for the treatment of painful menstruation, almost any type of internal hemorrhage, kidney stones, post-partum pains, abnormal uterine bleeding, abscesses and cancer of the lymphatic system. Externally, it is used in the treatment of diarrhea, tapeworms and injuries. An infusion of the root has also been used to treat gravel.

Narrowleaf Evening Primrose (*Oenothera biennis*). This plant is also known as sun drop or common evening primrose. CAUTION: Avoid if you are epileptic, schizophrenic or if you are on anticoagulants. Do not combine this plant with phenothiazines; it can trigger seizures, if taken on an empty stomach. This plant can be found in eastern North America (from Labrador to Texas and Florida). A poultice of the root has been used to treat piles and bruises and a tea made from the roots has also been used to treat obesity and bowel pains. The leaves and the bark have been used to treat whooping cough, gastro-intestinal issues and asthma. The essential oil has been used to treat rheumatoid arthritis, alcohol-related liver problems, eczema and fragile, breakable nails. It has also been used to treat hyperactivity, multiple sclerosis and pre-menstrual issues. Persistent and continual intake of the essential oil also helps to lower blood pressure and blood cholesterol levels.

Native Hemlock (*Tsuga*) This tree comes from the Pine family. But unlike the poison hemlock (conium), this species of Tsuga are not poisonous. This tree was used by Native Americans for making wooden items and baskets and as a dye for tanning hides. The pitch was usually applied as a salve or poultice to treat colds and to prevent sunburn. A decoction of the crushed bark was used to treat hemorrhages. The Forest Potawatomi and the Menominee Native Americans used the inner bark and twigs to brew a tea to treat fever, colds, flu, diarrhea and bladder and kidney problems. It was also used as a gargle for throat and mouth problems. Externally it was used to wash ulcers and sores.

Nevada jointfir (*Ephedra nevadensis*). The stem of this plant can be eaten raw or a tea made from the dried or fresh stems and used as medicine. The stems have also been used as a diuretic, fever reducer, blood purifier, tonic and as treatment for urogenital problems. The stems can be harvested at any time, dried and stored for later use. An infusion of this plant has been used to treat the first stages of syphilis, gonorrhea (any stage) and kidney problems. A poultice of the dried and crushed stems has also been used to treat sores. Note that Ephedra does not cure asthma but it is able to effectively alleviate asthma symptoms. Using this whole plant (as opposed to using isolated constituents of this plant such as ephedrine) is safer and rarely triggers any side-effects.

New England aster or Michaelmas daisy (*Symphyotrichum novae-angliae*). The Cherokee used a poultice of the roots of this plant for pain relief; sniffed the ooze of the roots to treat catarrh; and used an infusion of the roots for diarrhea. An infusion of the whole plant was also used for fever. The Iroquois used a decoction of the leaves and roots for fevers and weak skin. Some tribes also used this plant as a "love medicine". This plant can be found in Eastern North America.

Northern Pitch Pine (*Pinus rigida*). This herb is used to treat wounds, cuts, burns, sores, boils and rheumatism. It is also used as a laxative. A poultice of the plant is applied to boils to open them and also to treat abscesses. This plant has also been used to treat respiratory complaints (colds, coughs, tuberculosis and influenza, etc.) and to treat problems of the mucous membranes.

Northern red oak (*Quercus rubra*). The inner bark and bark of this tree have been found to be astringent, antiseptic, febrifuge (fever-reducing), emetic and tonic. The bark has tannins, which have been experimentally shown to be antiseptic, antiviral and anticancer but also carcinogenic. The northern red oak is used in the treatment of chronic dysentery, diarrhea, asthma, indigestion, hoarseness, severe coughs, intermittent fevers and bleeding etc. Externally, it is used as a skin wash for rashes, burns and skin eruptions. The bark is also masticated as a treatment for mouth sores. Galls produced on the tree are very astringent and can be used to treat chronic diarrhea, hemorrhages and dysentery etc. The northern red oak can be found around Eastern North America (from Nova Scotia to Georgia, west to Minnesota and Oklahoma).

Ohio horsemint, sunny woodmint (*Blephilia ciliate*). This herb is used to make a poultice to treat headaches. This plant can be found from Canada south to Georgia and west to Oklahoma.

Pacific beach strawberry (*Fragaria chiloensis*). This plant has astringent and antiseptic properties. It has been used to normalize the menstrual cycle. A poultice of the fresh leaves has been used for burns. The edible parts of this plant are the fruit which can be eaten raw or cooked. A tea can also be made from the leaves. This plant can be found near the coast all over South America and North America.

Pacific madrone (*Arbutus Menziesii*). The leaves and bark of this plant are astringent. The leaves can be used for the treatment of cramps, stomach ache and colds, etc. A poultice of the leaves can be applied to burns. An infusion of the bark has been used internally to treat diabetes mellitus and externally to treat cuts, sores and wounds. It has also been used as a gargle for sore throats. This plant can be found in Western North America (from British Columbia to California).

Pawpaw (*Asimina Triloba*). CAUTION: Pawpaw seeds contain a toxic alkaloid and are poisonous. Pawpaw leaves can cause contact dermatitis particularly in sensitive people. Nevertheless, pawpaw is used as a laxative. The leaves are diuretic. They are applied externally to ulcers, boils and abscesses. The seed contains the alkaline asininine, which is narcotic and causes vomiting. Pawpaw seeds have been powdered and applied to hair to eliminate lice. Pawpaw bark, although bitter, is used as a tonic. It has analobine, which is also used medicinally. Pawpaw can be found around South-eastern North America (from New Jersey to Florida, west to Texas and Nebraska).

Peach Leaved Willow (*Salix amygdaloides*). An infusion of the bark shavings from this plant has been used to treat diarrhea and other stomach ailments. A poultice of the bark has also been applied to mend bleeding cuts. A decoction of the branch tips has also been used to soak cramped legs and feet in for treatment. This plant can be found in North America (from British Columbia to New York, south to Texas).

Philadelphia Fleabane (*Erigeron philadelphicus*). CAUTION: This plant should not be taken by pregnant women as it can induce a miscarriage. Also contact with this plant can cause dermatitis in sensitive people. Nevertheless, tea made from this plant is used to treat gout, chronic diarrhea, gravel, menstrual problems and epilepsy. A poultice of the plant is used to treat headaches and is also applied on sores. Snuff made from the powdered florets of this plant is used to make a person with catarrh to sneeze. This plant can be found in North America (from Labrador to British Columbia, south to Florida and California).

Pitch Pine (*Pinus palustris*). This tree is also known as Southern Pine or Longleaf pine. CAUTION: The resins, wood and sawdust from this tree can trigger dermatitis in sensitive people. This tree can be found in south-eastern North America (from Virginia to Texas to Florida). The resin released from the pulpwood of this tree is often made into a vanillin flavoring and eaten as a condiment. The turpentine from the resin is used internally to treat of bladder and kidney ailments. It is also either ingested or used as a steam bath or rub to treat rheumatism. It is effective in treating respiratory complaints (such as coughs, tuberculosis, the flu) and diseases of the mucous membranes. It is also used externally to treat sores, wounds, boil, burns and various skin complaints. As an herb, it is administered in the form of teas/infusions, decoctions, poultices, liniments, inhalers and herbal steam baths. The turpentine from the resin was also used to treat chronic diarrhea and colic, to stop bleeding from the socket of the tooth, to de-worm and as a rubefacient.

Pokeweed (*Phytolacca americana*). This plant is also known as Poke. Pokeweed can be found and is native to the eastern United States. It is used to treat stomach ulcers, asthma, sores, boils, cramps and intestinal worms. It is also ingested as a spring tonic. Pokeweed has inhibitory effects on gram-negative and gram-positive bacteria and it is also parasiticidal.

Prairie sagewort (*Artemisia frigida*). CAUTION: Sensitive people should treat this plant with caution, as skin contact may possibly pose a danger of triggering dermatitis or other allergic reaction. Nevertheless, the leaves of this plant are used in the treatment of women's complaints. An infusion of the leaves is used in the treatment of indigestion, biliousness, colds and coughs. Juice from the masticated leaves are ingested to treat heartburn. A poultice of the crushed leaves has been applied to inflamed areas to lessen swelling. A hot poultice of the crushed leaves has also been applied to treat toothache. Prairie sagewort leaves have been placed in the nostrils to stop nosebleeds. The leaves have also been made into a sanitary towel and used to help lessen skin irritation. A tea of the leaves is also taken internally to treat irregular menstruation. The dried leaves have also been burnt as smudge to disinfect the home. A decoction made out of the roots has been used as a stimulant and a tonic. This plant can be found in North American (around Minnesota to Saskatchewan, Yukon, Texas and Arizona).

Rabbit tobacco (*Pseudognaphalium obtusifolium*). This plant is also called sweet everlasting. Rabbit tobacco is used along with other herb combinations to ease twitching, muscle cramps and muscle pain. An infusion of the plant is applied on nicks made over the area being treated and a poultice of the plant put over that area being treated. This plant, in conjunction with Carolina vetch, is ingested as treatment for rheumatism. A syrup made from the plant can be used to treat cough, while a decoction of the plant can be used to treat colds. The plant can also be liquidized and placed into the throat to treat diphtheria. It can also be chewed to treat sore throat/sore mouth and it can be smoked to treat asthma. This plant can be found in Eastern North America (from Ontario to Georgia and Alabama).

Ragweed (*Ambrosia trifida*). CAUTION: the pollen of this plant is a principal cause of hay fever in the USA. Ingesting or even making skin contact with ragweed can trigger allergic reactions in sensitive individuals. So, handle with caution and only under the supervision of a licensed doctor.

Nevertheless, the leaves have been applied externally to various skin complaints, including insect bites. Tea of ragweed leaves helps with treating nausea, pneumonia, fevers, intestinal cramps, mucous discharges and diarrhea. Also, juice from the withered leaves has been used to treat infected toes. And a tea of the roots has been used to treat menstrual disorders and stroke.

Rattlesnakemaster (*Eryngium aquaticum*). This plant is used mainly for the treatment of disorders of the kidneys and sexual organs. It has also been used as an antidote to snake venom. A poultice of the chewed roots is applied on the bite. The pounded roots are also used to promote the increased production of urine. And an infusion of the pounded roots is used to reduce fevers. This plant can be found around Eastern North America (New Jersey to Florida).

Red Osier Dogwood (*Cornus sericea*). Native Americans used the bark of this plant to treat fevers, diarrhea, skin problems etc. Drying the bark makes it less purgative. A decoction of the bark has been used in the treatment of headaches, coughs, diarrhea, colds and fevers. Externally, the decoction has also been used as a wash for sties, sore eyes and other infections. It has also been used to treat skin complaints such as rash, poison ivy and ulcers. The bark shavings have been applied as a dressing on wounds to stop bleeding. The plant is said to have been used to cure rabies-induced hydrophobia (fear of water).

Rocky Mountain Iris (*Iris missouriensis*). CAUTION: Many plants in this genus are assumed to be poisonous if ingested. Also this plant can trigger allergies and skin irritations in some people. So, caution is advised. Nevertheless, several North American Indian tribes have used this plant medicinally. An infusion of the root has been used in the treatment of bladder and kidney problems and stomach aches. A poultice of the crushed root is also placed in a cavity in the tooth or on the gum in order to bring toothache relief. A decoction of the root has been used as ear drops to treat earaches. A poultice of the mashed roots has also been used as a salve on venereal sores and applied on rheumatic joints for pain relief. A paste made from the ripe seeds has been used as a dressing for burns. This plant can be found around Western North American (from British Columbia to Mexico, east to South Dakota and Alberta).

Roundhead Lespedeza (*Lespedeza capitate*). An extract of this plant may be of benefit in chronic kidney disease. Experimentally, this plant has exhibited antitumor activity against carcinosarcoma. This plant is also apparently effective in lowering blood cholesterol levels. It is also believed to reduce blood nitrogen levels in persons with excessive levels of nitrogen in their urine. The root has been used as an antidote to poisoning. The stems have been used in the treatment of rheumatism and neuralgia. This plant can be found in North America (around Maine to Florida, west to Kansas and Texas).

Salmonberry (*Rubus spectabilis*). The root and leaves of this plant can shrink body tissues. A poultice made from the chewed leaves has been used as a dressing for burns. A decoction is used in the treatment of stomach problems. A decoction has also been used to ease labor pains. The powdered bark has been used to treat burns and sores. A poultice of the bark has also been applied to aching teeth and wounds to ease the pain. A poultice of the chewed bark has been used as a dressing to relive pain and clean wounds and burns. This plant can be found in Western North America (around Alaska to California and Texas).

Sassafras (*Sassafras albidum*). This plant is also called common sassafras or sassafras. CAUTION: The essential oil contains safrole, a carcinogenic. In large amounts, the essential oil of this plant is toxic, causing vomiting, dilated pupils, stupor, collapse and liver and kidney damage. If used on the skin, the oil may cause skin irritation in sensitive people. This plant can be found in eastern North America (from Maine to Ontario to Florida to Texas). The leaves of this tree are edible and can be eaten either cooked or raw (in salads or as soup thickener or as flavoring). The leaves are usually dried and ground into powder for future use. The powder is then consumed as tea or condiment. A tea can be made from the leaves, roots, root bark or flowers.

Sassafras is valued for its tonic effect on the body. A tea of the root bark of this plant is used as a blood purifier, a spring tonic and to treat rheumatism, kidney problems, skin eruptions, colds and gastrointestinal complaints. The pith from the twigs of this plant has been used (as a poultice, wash or ingested) to treat eye complaints, chest, kidney and liver problems. Sassafras has also been used to treat chicken pox, measles, influenza, colds and fever. Sassafras oil has been externally applied to treat lice infestation and to treat insect bites.

Native Americans used Sassafras in several ways: they drank a compound infusion of Sassafras roots and whisky as a remedy for the blood (blood medicine); to expel tape worms; to treat rheumatism; took an infusion or a decoction of the bark for "watery blood or to thin the blood or to clear the blood; Iroquois women took an infusion of the roots for post- childbirth fevers and cold; plant taken to treat high blood pressure, wounds, cuts, bruises, swellings, nosebleeds and as a wash for cataracts and sore eyes, and as a tonic.

Saw Palmetto (*Serenoa repens*). CAUTION: Avoid this plant if you are using hormonal drugs. Avoid during pregnancy and lactation. Take with food. Rare adverse effects include: gastrointestinal symptoms and mild headache. It may diminish libido in males and may increase blood pressure and the possibility of back pain. Saw palmetto berries are used to treat urinary tract problems and prostate problems. The berries also make a good tonic. The ripe (but partially dried fruit) has been used as an aphrodisiac, an expectorant, an antiseptic, a tonic, a diuretic and a sedative. Saw palmetto is taken internally to treat debility in elderly men, to treat impotence, absent or reduced sex drive, testicular atrophy, prostate enlargement, bronchial issues and wasting diseases. It is also used to stimulate breast enlargement in women. Saw palmetto also strengthens and builds body tissue and stimulates weight gain. A tincture or the fruit pulp is given to those suffering from general debility or wasting disease. The fruit also helps to strengthen the neck of the bladder, treat coughs, colds, asthma and irritated mucous membranes, etc. A suppository made of powdered saw palmetto fruits in cocoa butter, has been used as a vaginal and uterine tonic. This plant can be found around South-eastern North America, from South Carolina to Florida, west to Arkansas).

Scrub Pine (*Pinus virginiana*). This plant is also known as Jersey Pine or Virginia pine. CAUTION: The resins, wood and sawdust from this tree can trigger dermatitis in sensitive people. This tree can be found in eastern North America (from New York to Georgia to Alabama). The seed of this tree is edible and is eaten cooked or raw. The leaves are used to prepare a tea and resin released from the pulpwood of this tree is often made into a vanillin flavoring and eaten as a condiment. The turpentine from the resin is used internally to treat of bladder and kidney ailments. It is also either ingested or used as a steam bath or rub to treat rheumatism. It is effective in treating respiratory complaints (such as coughs, tuberculosis, the flu) and diseases of the mucous membranes. It is also used externally to treat sores, wounds, boil, burns and various skin complaints. As an herb, it is administered in the form of teas/infusions, decoctions, poultices, liniments, inhalers and herbal steam baths. An infusion made of the buds has been used as a dewormer and an infusion made of the plant's leaves has been used to treat high fevers.

The Choctaw drank an infusion of the buds of this tree to eliminate worms. The Rappahannock used the plant to treat kidney troubles.

The Cherokee put this pine to multiple uses. They used it to treat worms (they chewed the bark to eliminate worms); externally used the tree oil to wash painful joints; ingested a syrup made from the tree to treat rheumatism; used the oil or as steam or infusion to treat colds, measles and mumps; used in the form of a syrup by pregnant Cherokee women who had cough to treat the cough; used as a poultice to treat swollen breasts; a poultice made of the resin was used to treat tetterworm, scaldhead, ulcers and bruises; a compound infusion of the pine's needles was used by the Cherokee to bring out a fever; and as a laxative; as a sedative to treat hysterics; also used as a compound infusion to treat piles and to treat kidney complaints and a weak back; used as a tuberculosis remedy; syrup taken for chronic rheumatism and venereal disease; and the Cherokee used a syrup made from this pine as a poultice for swollen testicles caused by mumps.

Sheep Sorrel (*Rumex acetosella*). This plant is also known as common sheep sorrel. CAUTION: the leaves contain high levels of oxalic acid. Do not eat the leaves in large quantities. If you have arthritis, rheumatism, kidney stones, gout, or hyperacidity treat with caution. The root, leaves and seed of this plant are all edible. The leaves can be eaten cooked or raw but eat the leaves in small quantities only.

The leaves can be dried for future use. The root is eaten cooked. It can also be dried, ground into powder and used to make noodles. The seed can be eaten cooked or raw.

Sheep sorrel is detoxifying, mildly laxative, diuretic and good for treating gastrointestinal issues. A tea of the roots is used to treat excessive menstrual bleeding and diarrhea; while a tea of the leaves is used to treat inflammation, fevers, scurvy, kidney and urinary diseases. A poultice made from the leaves has been applied to cysts, tumors, and cancer. Indeed, sheep sorrel is included in the popular Essiac formula used for cancer treatment. This plant is also astringent. The Aleut applied a poultice of the steamed leaves to bruises and warts. The Cherokee used a poultice of the blossoms and leaves to treat old sores. The Mohegan chewed the fresh leaves to treat stomach ache, while the Squaxin ate the raw leaves to treat tuberculosis. The Anticosti, Cherokee, Hesquiat, Bella Coola, Hanaksiala, Delaware, Miwok, Saanich, Iroquois, Okanagan-Colville, Chehalis and the Thompson ate the tangy and tart leaves of this plant, fresh or boiled, as food.

Short-leaf Pine (*Pinus Echinata*). CAUTION: The resins, wood and sawdust can trigger dermatitis in sensitive people. This tree can be found in eastern North America (from New York to Texas and Florida). The resin released from this tree is often made into a vanillin flavoring and eaten as a condiment. The turpentine from the resin is used internally to treat of bladder and kidney ailments. It is also either ingested or used as a steam bath or rub to treat rheumatism. It is effective in treating respiratory complaints (such as coughs, tuberculosis, the flu) and diseases of the mucous membranes. It is also used externally to treat sores, wounds, boil, burns and various skin complaints. As an herb, the plant is administered in the form of teas/infusions, decoctions, poultices, liniments, inhalers and herbal steam baths. Tea made from the trunk pitch is used as a laxative. Also, tea made of the inner bark is used as an emetic, while a cold tea made of the plant's buds is used as a vermifuge (expels intestinal worms).

The Choctaw drank a cold infusion of the buds of this plant in order to deworm the stomach. The Nanticoke ingested pellets of the resin as a cathartic (stimulates an evacuation of the bowels, induces purging) and to treat soreness of the back. The Rappahannock took a decoction or a compound infusion of the top branches of this tree as a wash for swellings. And the Rappahannock also ingested a compound made of the dried, grated bark of this plant to induce vomiting.

Sitka Spruce (*Picea sitchensis*). Several Native American tribes have used this tree to treat lung complaints, sores, wounds etc. The inner bark of this tree is a laxative. It has been masticated and the juice swallowed for throat problems, colds and coughs. A decoction of the bark and branch tips has been used in the treatment of stomach pains, constipation, rheumatism and gonorrhea. A decoction of the cones has also been used to treat pain and rheumatism, back ache and gonorrhea. A poultice of the resin has been rubbed on rheumatic joints for relief. The resin has also been used as a poultice or a dressing on broken skin, cuts, wounds, boils, sores and infections. The resin has also been chewed to treat tuberculosis and as a breath freshener. Gum from the small branches and new shoots has been placed in the eyes to treat snow blindness. A decoction of the roots has also been used to treat diarrhea. This plant can be found around Western North America (from Alaska to North California).

Skunk Cabbage (*Symplocarpus Foetidus*). This plant contains calcium oxylate in all its parts, therefore, it is poisonous and should not be eaten raw. Note, however, that calcium oxylate is easily destroyed by thoroughly cooking or drying the plant. Nevertheless, handle this plant with care and only under the supervision of a licensed doctor. This plant has been used by the Winnebago Indian tribe and Dakota Indian tribe to stimulate the removal of phlegm in asthma and to treat nervous disorders, respiratory diseases, dropsy and rheumatism. Again, as the leaves and roots of this plant are toxic, they should not be eaten raw.

Slippery Elm (*Ulmus rubra*). CAUTION: Outer bark has caused abortions. Avoid, if pregnant. This tree can be found in central and southern North America (from Maine to Florida to Texas to North Dakota). The leaves, fruit and inner bark of this tree are edible. The leaves and the inner bark can be eaten cooked or raw. They can be dried, ground and powdered and used as a soup thickener or mixed with flour to make bread. The inner bark can also be used to prepare a tea. And the young fruit can be eaten cooked or raw.

Slippery elm bark is useful for treating chest mucous membrane irritations, stomach, intestinal and urinary issues and the tree is also included in the popular Essiac formula used for cancer treatment. The inner bark is used to treat sore throats, stomach ulcers, indigestion and digestive irritation. It has also been externally applied to burns, scalds and fresh wounds. The whole bark has been utilized as a mechanical irritant to cause abortions and so has now been banned in many countries.

The Cherokee took a decoction of the bark to ease labor; used the plant as a mild laxative and to treat "quinsies" and breast complaints; took a decoction of the inner bark for dysentery and stomach/bowel and heartburn issues in pregnant women; used a poultice of the inner bark for burn dressing, wounds and old sores; drank an infusion for catarrh, coughs and as a cold remedy; used a decoction of the bark as a wash for the eyes.

The Iroquois used a complex compound of this plant as a blood medicine to purify the blood; took a compound decoction to induce vomiting, weakness and sleepiness; used an infusion of the bark as a wash and as drops for sore eyes; took a decoction of bark to treat biliousness and to clean the stomach; took a compound decoction for parturition and to facilitate childbirth; took an infusion of the bark for dry birth; took a decoction of the bark for kidneys problems; smoked and exhaled the leaves for catarrh; used as a stimulant; chewed the raw bark to treat sore throats; and used a compound decoction as a poultice to treat swollen and infected tubercular glands.

The Alabama have used a decoction of the bark of slippery elm and gunpowder for delayed labor. They have also taken a decoction of the bark alone for prolonged labor. The Catawba have also used the bark to treat tuberculosis. The Chippewa gargled with a decoction of the bark or chewed the dried root to treat sore throat. The Dakota took a decoction of inner bark as a laxative. The Mahuna applied a poultice of the bark to broken and fractured limbs as an orthopedic aid. And the Menominee applied a poultice of the inner bark to draw pus out from a wound.

Spoonwood, calico-bush (*Kalmia latifolia*). This plant is used as an analgesic by placing an infusion of the leaves on nicks made over the location of the pain. The edges of 10 to 12 leaves are rubbed on the skin for rheumatism. The plant is also used as an infusion/wash to eliminate pests. A liniment made from the plant is also rubbed on affected areas to prevent cramps.

Spring onion, wild garlic. (*Allium tricoccum*). CAUTION: Although no information on toxicity of this species has been reported, there have been cases of poisoning after over-consumption of certain members of this genus, by some mammals. Dogs seem to be particularly susceptible. Nevertheless, this plant is eaten as food. The Cherokee have applied the warm juice of this plant to treat earaches. They have also ingested it as a spring tonic and they have also used it to treat croup. The

Iroquois have also used a decoction of this plant to treat worms in kids and as a spring tonic to detoxify the body. This plant can be found in Eastern North America (from Quebec, south to Virginia and Iowa).

Staggerbush, Piedmont staggerbush (*Lyonia mariana*). An infusion of the plant is used for foot ground-itch, toe itch and ulcers. This plant is native to the United States. It is listed as endangered in Pennsylvania, as historical in Rhode Island, and as a species of special concern in Connecticut.

Sweetflag (*Acorus calamus*). This plant is also called calamus. CAUTION: The fresh root of this plant can be poisonous. Do not use the isolated essential oil medicinally, as some forms of the plant may contain asarone, a potentially toxic carcinogenic. Avoid if you are on a monoamine oxidase inhibitor antidepressant. Also note the abortifacient effects of this plant's roots. An infusion of the root can cause an abortion. And only the root of this plant (but not the isolated essential oil) should be utilized in human herb therapy.

The leaves, stem and root are edible. The plant is also eaten as a condiment. Sweet flag is used mostly as a mild tonic and as a stimulant. It is useful in the treatment of convulsions, arthritis, dyspepsia, flatulence, epilepsy, diarrhea, and cancer, etc. It is also used internally to treat sinusitis, bronchitis, digestive complaints and anorexia nervosa. And it is also applied externally to treat neuralgia, rheumatic pains and skin eruptions. Chewing the root has been used to alleviate toothache and to eliminate the taste for tobacco. The root has also been used to treat flatulence, coughs, colds, bowel problems, colic, cholera, suppressed menses, dropsy, gravel, headache, sore throat, spasms, swellings, yellowish urine and heart disease.

Tansy (*Tanacetum vulgare*). CAUTION: This plant is poisonous if large quantities are ingested. The tea of this plant is presumably an abortifacient. There have also been fatality cases in North America caused by the drinking of strong brews of tea made from this plant. Nevertheless, the plant is used as a tonic and an infusion of the plant is used to treat backache.

Thinleaf huckleberry (*Vaccinium membranaceum*). An infusion of the stems and roots of this plant has been used in the treatment of arthritis, heart troubles and rheumatism. This plant can be found in Western North America (around Michigan and Alaska to California).

Turkey Rhubarb (*Rheum palmatum*). This plant is also called Chinese rhubarb and Da Huang. CAUTION: the leaves contain oxalic acid and are poisonous if consumed in large quantities. If you have arthritis, rheumatism, kidney stones, gout, or hyperacidity treat with caution. Avoid if you are pregnant, breastfeeding or have intestinal obstruction. Nevertheless, the leaf stem of the turkey rhubarb is edible, cooked or raw. Turkey rhubarb is good for digestive system issues. It is also one of the key ingredients of the Essiac anti-cancer tea formula. The roots can have a purgative or opposite effect depending on the quantity ingested. They can also be taken internally to treat gallbladder and liver complaints, diarrhea, chronic constipation, hemorrhoids, skin eruptions and menstrual problems. The root is used externally to treat burns.

Twinleaf (*Jeffersonia diphylla*). This plant is also called rheumatism root. An infusion of this plant has been used to treat dropsy, gravel and urinary tract complaints. A poultice of it has also been applied to treat sores and inflammation. The root of this plant contains berberine, which has been found to have anti-tumor properties. This plant can be found in Eastern North America (from New York and Ontario to Alabama and west to Wisconsin).

Upright prairie coneflower (*Ratibida columnifera*). The stem and leaves of this plant are analgesic. An infusion is used to treat headaches, fevers and stomach aches. A decoction of the plant is used as a wash for pain relief and to treat poison ivy rash. A decoction is also used as a sort of antidote to treat rattlesnake bites. This plant can be found in Western Northern America (from British Columbia to Montana, Nebraska, Texas, New Mexico and Mexico).

Virginia iris (*Iris virginica*). An infusion of the root of this plant has been used for the treatment of ailments of the liver. The root has also been pounded into a paste and used as a salve to treat skin problems. A decoction made from the root has also been used to treat cases of yellow urine.

Virginia Rose (*Rosa virginiana*). A decoction of the roots has been used as a bath and to treat worms in children. An infusion of the roots has also been drunk and used as a wash to treat bleeding cuts on the feet. An infusion of the roots has also been used as a wash to treat sore eyes. This plant is being investigated as a food that is capable of reducing the prevalence of cancer and also as a way of halting or reversing the metastasis of cancers. This plant can be found in Eastern North America (Newfoundland to Ontario, south to Louisiana).

Wild senna (*Senna hebecarpa*). This plant is also called American senna. The Cherokee have used an infusion of this plant to treat various ailments including: heart trouble, cramps and fever, etc. They have also used this plant to treat a condition they referred to as "blacks" (hands and eye sockets turn black) and they have also used the plant as a purgative. They used a compound decoction of this plant for a laxative. They used a compound infusion of this plant to treat pneumonia and fainting spells. And they used a poultice made from the root of to treat sores. The Iroquois also used the plant as a remedy for worms. This plant can be found in South-eastern North America (from Pennsylvania to Florida, Kansas and Iowa).

Willow Oak (*Quercus phellos*). This tree can be found in south-eastern North America (from Staten Island, New York to Georgia to Texas). The seeds of this tree are edible and eaten cooked. The seeds can be dried, ground, powdered and mixed with flours to make bread or used as thickening for stews. The seeds can also be roasted and consumed as a substitute for coffee. This tree produces galls that are very astringent and they have been used to treat chronic diarrhea, hemorrhages and dysentery. A decoction of the bark or wood chips has been used as an analgesic or a bath for cuts, sores, aches, pains and hemorrhoids. The Seminole externally applied a decoction of the bark or wood bits of this tree as an analgesic. Or they used it in a wash for cuts, aches and pains. The Seminole also used the willow oak as a dermatological aid to treat limb or back pains, sores, hemorrhoids or ballgame sickness. This tree is also used to treat bladder and kidney problems (including Bright's disease), diarrhea, viral infections, menstrual issues, sprains, swellings, sores and as a booster for other therapies. A decoction of the ashes of this tree was also placed on the tongue to cleanse the system.

Winged lythrum (*Lythrum alatum*). An infusion of this plant has been taken for kidney issues. This plant can be found in the wetland areas of central and eastern United States and Ontario.

Witherod, wild raisin (*Viburnum nudum*). An infusion of this plant has been taken to prevent recurrent spasms and also used as a wash for sore tongues. The root bark has been used as a diaphoretic and as a tonic. And the compound infusion has been taken for smallpox, fever and ague. This plant can be found in Eastern North America (from Maryland to Florida, west to Arkansas and Kentucky).

Yellow giant hyssop (*Agastache nepetoides*). A compound infusion of this plant is used as a wash for itch and poison ivy. This plant blooms from July to September. It can be found from Southern Canada to southeastern United States.

Yerba Mansa (*Anemopsis californica*). Several Native American tribes have used Yerba mansa to treat different medical complaints. An infusion of the plant is used to bathe aching muscles and sore feet. The root is chewed for issues with the mucous membrane. A tea made from the root is used as a blood purifier, as a treatment for menstrual cramps, syphilis, gonorrhea, pleurisy and as a general pain remedy. An infusion of the plant is used to treat chest congestion, colds and stomach ulcers. The dried and powdered plant has been used as a disinfectant on wounds. The fresh moist leaves have been used as a salve or poultice on cuts, burns and wounds. And an infusion of the bark has been used as a wash for open sores. This plant is found around South-western North America (from California to Mexico).

CHAPTER 3: THE LEADING DISEASE-CAUSES OF DEATH IN THE USA AND THEIR NATIVE-AMERICAN HERBAL CURES AND REMEDIES

Heart disease

Heart disease is the No. 1 killer disease in the American society. Many nutrients in Native American foods good quality fats and flavonoids (plant pigments protective of cardiovascular disease and vascular degeneration, etc.) which are known to reduce the risk of heart disease.

Hawthorn berry. (*Crataegus laevigata and Crataegus douglasii*). The flower, leaf and berry of this plant are all medicinal. Native Americans ingested a decoction of the bark of this plant to treat stomach problems, venereal disease and diarrhea. They also took hawthorn to thin the blood and strengthen the heart. Hawthorn tones the blood and strengthens the heart. It is also used for several cardiovascular disorders. Hawthorn increases the heart's ability to contract and relaxes the outer blood vessels so that the heart has less resistance to work against. Hawthorn also relaxes the coronary-artery walls and lets more blood to flow into heart cells. Hawthorn helps to balance the blood pressure and relieves conditions such as heart pain or angina. Hawthorn also helps to treat or prevent atherosclerosis which contributes to heart attacks and angina. Flavonoids in hawthorn also help to strengthen and protect the cardiovascular tissue.

Sassafras (*Sassafras albidum*). Sassafras was used to treat measles, chicken pox, colds, flu, fever, a blood purifier, a spring tonic and a general heart tonic FOR GENERAL HEART HEALTH.

Sweetflag or calamus (*Acorus calamus*). The root was used to treat flatulence, colds, coughs, bowel problems, colic, cholera, suppressed menses, dropsy, gravel, headache, sore throat, spasms, swellings, and yellowish urine AND HEART DISEASE.

American hemp, dogbane. (*Apocynum androsaemifolium*). This plant was used by the Prairie Potawatomis AS A HEART MEDICINE. The fruit was boiled when it was still green, and the resulting decoction drunk. It was also used for kidney problems and for dropsy.

Purslane (*Portulaca Oleracea*). Purslane is a great source of the antioxidant vitamins A, C, and E. It also contains riboflavin, calcium, phosphorus, magnesium, and iron. It is also the richest known plant source of omega-3 fatty acids which may help REDUCE THE RISK OF HEART DISEASE. It does this by lowering cholesterol and blood pressure and by reducing the tendency of the blood to form clots in the arteries. It was used to reduce the risk of heart disease.

Rosehips (*Rosa canina.)* All parts of this plant are used for physical and spiritual medicine. A tea from rosehips is prepared for sore throats, colds, diarrhea and other conditions when an astringent is helpful. Rose hips are high in Vitamin C and bioflavonoids Rose hips were used to boost immunity and for PROTECTING THE HEART AND THE BLOOD VESSELS.

White willow (*Salix alba*). Willow is a rich source of a compound called salicin, which is very similar to the painkilling, fever-reducing ingredient in aspirin. Willow is heart-protective and was used by Native Americans to protect against heart disease. Just like aspirin, willow substantially REDUCES THE RISK OF HEART ATTACKS and strokes. It also inhibits the formation of blood clots that can potentially block arteries and prevent blood from reaching the heart or brain. One cup of willow bark tea every other day is okay. But just like aspirin, it may also irritate the stomach. Also, willow should not be given to children as it may elevate the possibility of Reye's syndrome.

Red clover (*Trifolium pratense*). Native Americans used this plant to treat respiratory conditions and inflammation. But recent studies have found that red clover is PREVENTIVE AND PROTECTIVE OF HEART DISEASE. It does this by improving circulation and lowering cholesterol.

Violet Prairieclover (*Dalea purpurea*). This plant has been used by the Chippewa Indians as a HEART

MEDICINE. A decoction of the blossoms and leaves are INGESTED FOR HEART HEALTH.

Cancer

Cancer is the second leading cause of mortality in the United States. In 2017, for example, the total number of cancer deaths in the United States was 599,108. The percentage of cancer deaths of total deaths in 2017 in the United States was 21.3%. The three leading causes of cancer-death among American males are: first, lung and bronchial cancer; second, prostate cancer; and third, colorectal cancer. Among American females, the three leading causes of cancer-death are: first, lung and bronchial cancer; second, breast cancer; and third, colorectal cancer.

Conventional medicine has several approaches to treating cancer including: chemotherapy, hormone therapy, immunotherapy, personalized medicine or precision medicine (using genetic testing), radiation therapy, stem cell transplant, targeted therapies (e.g., monoclonal antibodies and small molecule drugs) and surgery. But what about herbal remedies? Do Native American Indians possess any (yet unexplored) therapeutic cancer secrets that might benefit those who wish to pursue an herbal and natural course of treatment to cure cancer? Or any such secrets that might benefit those who wish to prevent cancer via natural, herbal means? Well let's take a look.

Creosote bush (*Larrea tridentata*). This plant was used in traditional Native American medicine to treat several illnesses and diseases including respiratory disorders. But today, modern scientific research has shown that creosote bush can also be used to effectively treat cancer and many viral diseases. Apparently, creosote bush has the capacity to penetrate a virus' envelope and nucleus in order to thwart vital viral genetic functions. Indeed, one compound isolated from the creosote bush (called, NDGA or nordihydroguaiaretic acid) has been demonstrated in clinical studies to inhibit cancerous growth. Creosote Bush should be used with care as it has very serious side effects and should be eaten or used only under the supervision of a doctor. Under the supervision of a licensed doctor, the flower buds of creosote bush are usually pickled in vinegar and eaten. Tea can also be made out of the stem and leaves and drank. The twigs may also be chewed.

Greater Burdock (*Arctium lappa*). An ingredient (arctigenin) in the plant, greater burdock, blocks cancer growth. Greater burdock is anti-inflammatory, antiviral and with a mucilage content. Chinese researchers have found that the burdock compound, arctigenin, suppresses cancer growth. The researchers found that arctigenin arrests the proliferation of cancer cells, prevents their migration to other parts of the body and stops the development of tumors. In animal studies, arctigenin produced a cellular genetic change that led to the suppression of tumor growth (by 70%); and a suppression in the growth of prostate cancer cells (by 75%). These studies have been noted to have good promise of being eventually applied to human cases.

Japanese researchers have also found that arctigenin from Greater Burdock is active against lung cancer cells. And South Korean researchers have also found that arctigenin also significantly halted the metastasis of human breast cancer cells. Indeed, it has been found that greater burdock's arctigenin (a cancer-specific phytochemical) has one of the highest levels of anti-cancer potentialities among many comparable herbs; and that arctigenin is partly responsible for the tumor-killing capacity found in herbal medicine. Arctigenin kills human lung cancer cells, human stomach cancer cells and human liver cancer cells. Note that greater burdock is also one of the key ingredients of the Essiac anti-cancer tea formula.

Greater celandine (*Chelidonium majus*). Greater celandine is a toxic plant. It is generally not recommended for internal use unless under strict supervision of a licensed doctor. It has been used in traditional native American medicine. Modern research findings now propose that the plant has anti-cancer capacity and that it destroys cancer cells via apoptosis.

Cancer root (*Orobanche fasciculate*). There are species of this plant (cancer root) that are parasitic on the roots of sweet sage. These forms of cancer root have been used as a treatment for cancer. Additionally, powdered and dried cancer root has been inserted into the rectum as treatment for hemorrhoids. The plant, cancer root (as a whole) is edible and can be eaten cooked or raw. To date, there are no known hazards of this plant.

Cancer weed (*Salvia lyrata*). This plant has been reported as a folk remedy for cancer. Additionally, the leaves, root and seeds can be made into an ointment or salve for the treatment of sores and wounds. Fresh leaves of cancer weed can be applied to remove warts. To date, there are no known hazards of this plant.

Red clover (*Trifolium pratense*). This plant has been used by the Shinnecock Indians to treat cancer. The powdered plant is mixed in boiling water and taken for stomach cancer.

Western larch (*Larix occidentalis*). The Thompson Indians used this plant to treat cancer in the following ways. (i) A decoction of the tops of the plant were used to clean and wash the areas of the body affected by cancer. (ii) And a decoction of small branch pieces from the plant were ingested, internally to treat the cancer. This treatment would cause a cancer patient to recover and to regain weight.

Indian pokeroot (*Phytolacca decandra*). Indian pokeroot has been used for the treatment of cancer of any kind.

Bloodroot (*Sanguinaria canadensis*). Bloodroot is a very poisonous plant, an emetic and a laxative. But it has also been used to treat cancers.

White willow (*Salix alba*). The bark of white willow is an astringent, expectorant, hemostatic, and a tonic. This plant has also been used to treat cancers.

Sheep sorrel (*Acetosella vulgaris*). Sheep sorrel has also been taken for incipient cancers.

Goldenseal (*Hydrastis Canadensis*). Goldenseal has also been used for the treatment of cancer.

Chishima zasa (*Sasa kurilensis*). A possible cure for cancer has been discovered residing inside the leaf of this plant.

Desert thorn (*Lycium fremontii*). This plant is being studied for its capacity to reduce the occurrence of cancer and also as a viable agent for arresting, reversing or retarding the advancement of cancer. CAUTION: There are no known records of toxicity for this particular species, but caution still needs to be observed because this species comes from a botanical family that includes many poisonous plants. So, handle even this particular species (particularly its unripe fruits and leaves) with caution and only under the supervision of a licensed doctor.

Hound's tongue (*Cynoglossum officinale*). Hound's tongue contains allantoin, a highly effective agent that speeds up the healing process in the body. This plant also has a wide antitumor reputation for cancers of various types. It has also been used as a pain reliever. CAUTION. While hound's tongue has been used in the treatment of cancer, it can also be carcinogenic (if taken internally, in large doses).

Akebia (*Akebia quinata*). The edible parts of this plant include the fruit and the leaves (often prepared as tea). This plant has been used internally for the control of fungal and bacterial infections and for the treatment of amenorrhea (absent menstruation), also to improve lactation, and for urinary tract infections. Akebia is a well-known remedy for cancer.

Chronic Lower Respiratory Diseases (Chronic Bronchitis, Emphysema and Asthma)

CLRD refers to a group of certain conditions of the lung characterized by a blockage of airflow causing shortness of breath and other breathing-related difficulties. These CLRD diseases include: chronic bronchitis; emphysema; and asthma. Chronic Lower Respiratory Diseases (CLRD), as a group, is the third leading cause of mortality in the United States. In 2017, for example, the total number of CLRD deaths in the United States was 160,201, representing 5.7% of the total deaths in the United States in 2017. And one disturbing fact about CLRD is that while mortality rates for the top two causes of death in the US (heart disease and cancer) are decreasing, the mortality rates from CLRD are continuing to rise.

Tobacco smoking is largely the most significant risk factor for chronic bronchitis and emphysema. Indeed, tobacco smoking accounts for approximately 80% of all chronic bronchitis and emphysema cases. As for asthma, the cause appears to be genetic, while tobacco smoking (including secondhand smoking) aggravates the condition.

Conventional medicine has several approaches to treating CLRD. For chronic bronchitis and emphysema, the treatment approaches include:

(i) cessation of tobacco smoking (including avoidance of exposure to secondhand smoke);
(ii) avoidance of occupational exposures;
(iii) avoidance of other outdoor and indoor pollutants;
(iv) pulmonary rehabilitation via exercises to decrease symptoms, enhance quality of life, and increase emotional and physical participation in daily activities;
(v) medications (although to date, there is no alterative medication for chronic bronchitis and emphysema). However, drugs such as bronchodilators, inhaled corticosteroids, antibiotics are the most commonly used medications in treating chronic bronchitis and emphysema. These drugs help to reduce swelling, inflammation and mucus production. Pneumococcal and influenza vaccines are also helpful in tampering mortality among COPD patients.
(vi) Oxygen Therapy is often only introduced in severe cases of chronic bronchitis or emphysema or where there is pulmonary hypertension or congestive heart failure.
(vii) And surgery. Surgical procedures are usually limited to a bullectomy or a lung volume reduction surgery or a lung transplantation.
(ix) As for asthma, conventional medical treatment typically involves the use of bronchodilators, cessation of tobacco smoking, avoidance of exposure to secondhand smoke and the avoidance of asthma triggers (which is the most effective method of

controlling asthma). Triggers vary from person to person and include dissimilar things such as cockroaches, feathers or cold air, etc.

And what about herbal medicine? Does Native American herbology have any more secrets to offer with regard to CLRD, chronic bronchitis, emphysema, asthma and pulmonary distress and respiratory conditions in general? Again, let's review the evidence.

Common Yarrow (*Achillea millefolium*). This plant has been used by the Bella Coola Native American tribe as a pediatric pulmonary and respiratory aid. A poultice of yarrow leaves combined with eulachon grease has been applied to the back and chest of children to treat bronchitis.

Brewer's Angelica (*Angelica breweri*). This herb has been used by the Native American Washo tribe as a respiratory aid. An infusion of the dried and scraped root was taken for bronchitis.

Forked Sagewort (*Artemisia furcate*). Forked Sagewort was used by the Mendocina Native American tribe as a respiratory aid. A decoction of the leaves of this plant was taken internally for bronchitis.

Big Sagebrush (*Artemisia tridentate*). This herb was used by the Diegueno Native American tribe as a respiratory aid, cold remedy and cough medicine. An infusion of the dried or fresh leaves of the herb is ingested to treat a serious cold accompanied by coughing and bronchitis.

Curlycup Gumweed (*Grindelia squarrosa*). Curlycup gumweed was used by the Crow and the Flathead Native American tribes as a respiratory aid. The herb was taken as treatment for asthma and bronchitis.

Carrotleaf Biscuitroot (*Lomatium dissectum*), The Paiute, Shoshoni, Great Basin and Washo Native American tribes used this herb as a respiratory aid. A decocotion of the dried root was taken for bronchitis, pneumonia and hayfever. Also a compound of roots of this plant was used as herbal steam for nasal congestion, lung congestion and asthma. Sometimes the pulverized roots of this plant were also smoked alone or in compound for the treatment of asthma

Indian Walnut (*Aleurites moluccana*). The Hawaiians used the Indian walnut as a respiratory aid. They combined the bark of this plant with other plants and pounded them together. The resulting liquid was heated and drank as a treatment for asthma.

Indianhemp (*Apocynum cannabinum*)
American Spikenard (*Aralia racemose*)
Stinking Chamomile (*Anthemis cotula*)
Horseradish (*Armoracia rusticana*)
Licorice Bedstraw (*Galium circaezans*)
Cultivated Licorice (Glycyrrhiza glabra)
Man of The Earth (*Ipomoea pandurate*)
Meadow Garlic (*Allium canadense*),
Cultivated Garlic (*Allium sativum*) and

Wild Garlic (*Allium vineale*) were all used by the Native American Cherokee tribe as respiratory aids for the treatment of asthma.

Hyssop (*Hyssopus officinalis*). The Native American Cherokee tribe also used this plant as a respiratory and pulmonary aid. It was made into a syrup and taken internally for asthma, lung diseases and breast diseases.

Elecampane Inula (*Inula helenium*). The Cherokee also used this plant as a respiratory aid. The root was used aa decoction and taken internally for asthma.

Oahu Wormwood (*Artemisia australis*) was used by the Hawaiians as a reproductive aid. The leaves were used in the preparation of asthma medicine.

Olapa (*Cheirodendron gaudicchaudii*). The Hawaiins also used this plant as a respiratory aid. The root bark and other plants were pounded and squeezed and the resulting liquid taken for asthma.

Elecampane Inula (*Inula helenium*). The Iroquois Native American tribe used this plant as a pediatric aid and a respiratory aid. An infusion of the dried leaves was given to children for asthma. An infusion of the roots was also taken internally by adults for asthma.

Common Juniper (*Juniperus communis*). This plant was taken by the Chippewa Native Indian Tribe as a respiratory aid. The leaves and twigs were made into a decoction that was taken for asthma.

California Sycamore (*Platanus racemose*). The Diegueno Native American tribe used this plant as a respiratory aid. A decoction of the bark was taken for a week for a week for asthma

Grand Fir (*Abies grandis*). This plant was used by the Gitksan Native American tribe as pulmonary aid. A poultice of compound containing the bark of the plant was used as a chest plaster for lung hemorrhage.

Subalpine Fir (*Abies lasiocarpa)*. This plant was used by the Blackfoot and Montana Native American tribes as a pulmonary aid. The gummy secretions from the bark were taken internally for lung troubles.

Calamus (*Acorus calamus*). The Micmac Native American tribe used this plant as a pulmonary aid. They used the root for the treatment of lung ailments, pleurisy and pneumonia.

Red Baneberry (*Actaea rubra*). The Thompson Native American tribe used this plant as a pulmonary aid. A decoction of the plant was taken for bronchial or lung problems. The Blackfoot took a decoction of the roots of this plant to treat coughs and colds.

White Colicroot (*Aletris farinose*). The Cherokee Native American tribe took this plant as a pulmonary aid, as treatment for lung diseases, tuberculosis and as a cough medicine.

Scarlet Indian Paintbrush (*Castilleja miniata*). The Gitksan Native American tribe used this plant as an anti-hemorrhagic. A decoction of the whole plant was taken internally for bleeding or stiff lungs, sore eyes and lame back. A decoction of seeds was taken for coughs.

Stroke and Cerebrovascular Diseases

White willow (*Salix*). Willow is a rich source of a compound called salicin, which is very similar to the painkilling, fever-reducing ingredient in aspirin. Willow is heart protective and was used by Native Americans to protect against heart disease and STROKES. Just like aspirin, it also inhibits the formation of blood clots that can potentially block arteries and prevent blood from reaching the heart or brain. Willow also, substantially reduces the risk of heart attacks and STROKES. One cup of willow bark tea every other day is okay. But just like aspirin, it may also irritate the stomach. And it should not be given to children as it may increase the danger of Reye's syndrome.

Bilberry (*Vaccinium myrtillus*). Bilberry extract is used to treat or prevent fragile capillaries. Fragile capillaries can lead to blood or fluid leaking into tissues. This could further trigger a STROKE, heart attack, hemorrhage or blindness. Bilberry is able to protect capillaries via its ability to increase the flexibility of red blood cell membranes. This action allows capillaries to stretch, increasing blood flow, and red blood cells can deform into a shape that eases their way through narrow capillaries. So, billberry is protective against STROKE.

Anti-high blood pressure herbal group. Many of the herbs that Native Americans used all the time (e.g. black cohosh, garlic, onions, ginseng, plantain, purslane, saw palmetto, corn, honeysuckle, hawthorn, and yarrow, are now known to lower blood pressure. And when blood pressure is low, the risk for STROKE is lowered, too. So the anti-high blood pressure herbal groups mentioned above was used as protective for STROKE.

Anti-cholesterol, anti-blood clotting, anti-stroke herbal group. The accumulation of cholesterol in the blood vessels can lead to the development of blood clots. And blood clots can cause STROKES. It therefore follows that any treatment that reduces cholesterol also reduce your chances of developing blood clots. Hawthorn, motherwort, ginkgo, bilberry, evening primrose oil, garlic, onion, cayenne, lemongrass, turmeric and ginger all reduce cholesterol and blood clots. Now, here's an anti-cholesterol, anti-blood clotting, anti-stroke tonic for you. Mix 2 teaspoons of hawthorn flowers; 1 teaspoon of motherwort leaves; 1 teaspoon of ginkgo leaves; 1 teaspoon of ginger rhizome. Steep in hot water for five minutes. Strain and drink from time to time and you're good to go! In other words, the anti-cholesterol, anti-blood clotting, anti-stroke herbal group was used as protective for STROKE.

Annual Ragweed (*Ambrosia artemisiifolia*). The Iroquois Native American tribe used this plant as a heart medicine. An infusion of the roots was taken internally for stroke.

Wild Strawberry (*Fragaria sp.*) The Iroquois also used this plant as a heart medicine. A compound of it was taken to treat stroke.

Western Pearlyeverlasting (*Anaphalis margaritacea*). The Ojibwa Native American tribe sprinkled the powdered flowers of this plant on coals and inhaled the smoke to revive stroke victims.

Elecampane Inula (*Inula helenium*). The Iroquois also took this plant as a heart medicine. The decoction of the roots of the plant was taken for stroke.

American Skunkcabbage (*Lysichiton americanus*). The Tolowa and the Yurok Native American tribes used the roots of this plant in a steam to treat stroke.

Alzheimer's Disease

Alzheimer's disease is the fifth leading disease cause of mortality in the United States. In 2017, for example, the total number of Alzheimer's deaths in the United States was 121,404, representing 4.3% of the total deaths in the United States in 2017. According to the Alzheimer's Association, in the United States, about 5.8 million people have Alzheimer's disease, and by 2050, this number is expected to increase to about 14 million people. And, unfortunately, Alzheimer's disease is the only one of the top ten disease causes of mortality in the United States, that cannot be slowed, prevented or cured. Alzheimer's disease causes neurons to deteriorate and die. It is the most frequent cause of dementia which is a gradual degeneration of mental functions and behavioral capabilities that disorders a person's ability to manage themselves autonomously and unaided.

There is no cure for Alzheimer's disease or any treatment that alters the disease process in the brain. Gradual and worsening memory loss, problems with thinking and reasoning and problems with making judgments and decisions, problems with planning and performing familiar tasks, changes in personality and behavior, are all principal signs and symptoms of Alzheimer's disease. The exact causes of Alzheimer's disease aren't fully understood but it is believed that the disease is caused by a combination of genetic, environmental and lifestyle factors that affect the brain in the long term. Researchers, however, have found that Beta-amyloid proteins can cluster together (along with other cellular debris) and form plaques in the brain which disrupt cell-to-cell communication and ultimately has a toxic effect on brain cells. Researchers have also found that tau proteins (which help to support and supply nutrients to brain cells) change shape in Alzheimer's disease and agglomerate as structures called neurofibrillary tangles which disrupt the neural transport system and are also ultimately toxic to cells.

Here are some herbs that can be very helpful in treating Alzheimer's disease:

Celery seeds (*Apium graveolens*). The Houma Native American tribe used wild celery as a tuberculosis remedy. They took a compound decoction of the plant along with whiskey to treat tuberculosis. But modern scientific research has now found that celery seed (from either wild celery or cultivated celery) slows Alzheimer's Disease, reduces brain injury and possesses memory and cognitive benefits. The L-3-n-butylphthalide (L-NBP) (an extract from celery seed) inhibits brain injury and oxidation, while increasing cognition and memory. Thus celery seed extract may be a treatment to prevent and possibly reverse Alzheimer's disease. The extract blocks the tau protein phosphorylation and prevents and reduces amyloid-beta plaque build-up. Celery seeds also contain significant antioxidants, and increase vascular circulation which is important for brain health.

Rosemary (*Rosmarinus officinalis*). Indeed, rosemary emulates Aricept (sold generically as donepezil). Aricept is the No. 1 synthetic drug therapy for Alzheimer's disease. Aricept treats Alzheimer's by preventing the breakdown of acetylcholine. Rosemary does the same thing (albeit naturally). Indeed, Aricept contains only a single unnatural and synthetic AChE inhibitor, while rosemary contains nearly a dozen, natural AChE (acetylcholine esterase) inhibitors that prevent the breakdown of ACh (acetylcholine). In Alzheimer's, there is a shortage of acetylcholine, so we want to inhibit (or block) a compound (esterase) that removes the little acetylcholine in the brain so that more of the acetylcholine can stay in the brain.

Consuming Aricept or rosemary will block the esterase and boost acetylcholine. Thus rosemary fights Alzheimer's disease, dementia and strengthens memory. Rosemary shampoo, herbal tea, skin lotions and bath solutions are pleasant and safe ways to reduce the risk of Alzheimer's disease and retard dementia.

Turmeric (*Curcuma longa*). Turmeric spice contains curcumin. Native Hawaiians used this plant as a blood medicine and a nose medicine. The shoots, bulbs and other plants were pounded and squeezed resulting in liquid taken internally to cleanse the blood and also used as a gargle. The resulting liquid fumes were also inhaled to treat nose growths, nose troubles and odors. Modern medical research has also shown that the plant has properties that will significantly boost the memory and improve mood in those with age-related memory loss, despite aging. It has also been found that turmeric (curcumin) has anti-inflammatory and antioxidant properties, reduces brain inflammation (which is linked to Alzheimer's disease and depression) significantly boosts attention and memory abilities, and mild improvements in mood, and significantly reduces amyloid and tau signals in the amygdala and hypothalamus regions of the brain. The hypothalamus and amygdala are regions of the brain that control several emotional and memory functions. Thus taking turmeric (curcumin) could provide meaningful cognitive benefits over the long term. Side effects may include abdominal pain and nausea.

Greater burdock (*Arctium lappa*). An ingredient (arctigenin) in the plant, Greater Burdock, significantly boosts cognition and memory and blocks cancer growth. Greater Burdock is anti-inflammatory, antiviral and with a mucilage content. It is often used for lung and skin infections and to soothe mucosal membranes. Chinese researchers have found that the burdock compound, arctigenin, suppresses the production of the beta-amyloid protein that characteristically occurs in Alzheimer's disease. It was also found that arctigenin significantly improves functional activity cognition and memory and produces a 62% to 73% reduction in memory deficits. They found that the two major ingredients in Greater burdock (arctigenin and arctiin) produce these results by inhibiting acetylcholinesterase (which degrades acetylcholine), which then allows acetylcholine (an important neurotransmitter) to flourish, thus allowing better communication between brain/nerve cells. So, Greater Burdock helps with memory and cognition and with Alzheimer's disease and dementia.

American ginseng (*Panax quinquefolius*). The Menominee Native American tribe have used this plant as a psychological and mental aid. Specifically, they used this plant as a tonic for strengthening mental powers.

Beggarslice (*Hackelia virginiana*) The Cherokee used this plant for good memory

Mediterranean diet. By the way, researchers at Harvard University have found that the

Mediterranean diet benefits Alzheimer's disease and slows aging decline in cognition. The Mediterranean diet consists of a high-consumption of fruits, legumes, vegetables, fish, cereals and monounsaturated fatty acids (e.g. olive oil) and a low consumption of meat, poultry, dairy products, moderate amounts of alcohol and saturated fatty acids. Indeed, a Mediterranean diet supplemented with either extra virgin olive or nuts results in about a 66% decrease in the risk of mild cognitive impairment (MCI) and thus Alzheimer's disease. Olive oil is a prevalent ingredient in the Mediterranean diet. And olive oil is among the healthiest oils because it contains a number of medicinal phytonutrients including tyrosol, hydroxytyrosol, verbascoside and oleuropein (an antioxidant and anticancer agent that also reduces inflammation and blood pressure). Indeed, other research has found that the consumption of increased measures of olive oil gives rise to a 15% decline in verbal fluency and a 17% decrease in overall cognitive decline

Furthermore, the Mediterranean diet helps to prevent Alzheimer's disease, even more so than multivitamin supplements. Indeed, besides vitamin E, other supplements have failed to demonstrate any benefit to, or capacity to prevent Alzheimer's disease (but exercise and diet do). In any event it is important to note that ingesting more than 400 international units (IU) of Vitamin E per day is dangerous for individuals with a risk for cardiovascular disease or the active disease itself. The bottom line, anyway, is that greater compliance with the Mediterranean diet is linked to a significantly reduced cognitive decline and a reduced risk of Alzheimer disease.

Lemon balm(*Melissa officinalis*). It has been found that aromatherapy and massage can help people with dementia to relax, improve their cognition and, generally, help to treat or prevent dementia. Lemon balm (which may be used in aromatherapy and/or massage) has been specifically identified as being especially beneficial to the treatment of Alzheimer's disease. Lemon balm has been identified as useful for the improvement of memory, cognition and mood in the treatment of Alzheimer's disease. On the other hand, lavender oil has also been identified as having the capacity to reduce incidents of belligerent behavior in dementia. The essential oil, extract and tea of lemon balm are used in traditional and in alternative medicine (including aromatherapy).

Person-centric care. Dementia's natural treatment among Native Americans was to simply engage the loved one suffering from dementia, spend time with them and provide them with the necessary stimulus. In other words, the Native American response to dementia was to provide understanding, patience, attention, care and love to the person suffering from dementia. Engagement and stimulation can be achieved by referencing old thoughts and events, pleasant childhood memories, playing the music and games that they once loved or engaging in any other effective memory-jogging activity.

You may note that the above approach is similar to the person-centered approach to dementia treatment that is advocated today by the Alzheimer's Society. The key points of that person-centered care include: treating the person with respect and dignity; understanding their interests and hobbies, likes and dislikes; understanding their point-of-view, culture, history and lifestyle; providing conversation and relationship opportunities to the person; keeping the person active and varying their everyday experiences; and involving the person in the developing of a care plan for them. This person-centered approach works.

Preventing Alzheimer's disease. Evidence suggests that heart-healthy (cardiovascular-healthy) lifestyle choices may lower your risk of developing Alzheimer's disease and other causes of dementia. These lifestyle choices include the following: exercise regularly; eat fresh produce, healthy oils and foods low in saturated fats; manage your blood pressure, cholesterol levels and diabetes; quit smoking or don't start smoking; and participate in events that require mental and social engagement.

Diabetes

Diabetes is the sixth leading disease cause of mortality in the United States. In 2017, for example, the total number of diabetes deaths in the United States was 80,058 representing 2.9% of the total deaths in the United States in 2017. Type 1 diabetes occurs when a person's pancreas cannot produce enough insulin. This type of diabetes is common where there is already a specific genetic disposition to the disease or where there is a family history of the disease or in children that are between 4 years and 7 years of age or in people that reside in climates that are far from the equator. Type 2 diabetes occurs when a person's body does not make enough insulin to control blood sugar levels or when a person's body becomes resistant to insulin. Type 2 diabetes is more common among people who are obese or overweight; people with a history of diabetes in their family and people who are 45 years of age or older. Diabetes can lead to serious health complications, including heart disease, blindness, kidney failure and a possibility of the limbs being amputated.

Now let's review some of the anti-diabetes herbs and remedies from Native American herbology.

Calamus (*Acorus calamus*). This plant has been used by the Lakota Native American tribe as a diabetes remedy. An infusion of the roots was taken internally for diabetes.

Yerba Mansa (*Anemopsis californica*). The Kawaiisu Native American tribe took this herb for diabetes. A decoction of the crushed roots was taken internally for diabetes.

Wild Sarsaparilla (*Aralia nudicaulis*). This herb was used by the Iroquois Native American tribe for the treatment of sugar diabetes.

American Spikenard (*Aralia racemose*). The American Spikenard was used by the Algonquin Native American tribe of Quebec as a diabetes remedy. An infusion of the chopped roots and spurge were taken for sugar diabetes.

Pacific Madrone (*Arbutus menziesii*). This herb was used by the Cowichan Native American tribe as a diabetes remedy. An infusion of the bark was drunk for diabetes.

Horseradish (*Armoracia rusticana*). The Iroquois Native American tribe also used this plant as a remedy for sugar diabetes.

Alaska Sagebrush (*Artemisia alaskana*).
Boreal Sagebrush (*Artemisia arctica*).
Fringed Sagewort (*Artemisia frigida*).
These plants were all independently used by the Tanana Native American tribe as remedies for diabetes. A decoction of any of these plants was taken internally for diabetes.

New Jersey tea (*Ceanothus americanus*).
Sweet woodreed (*Cinna arundinacea*).
These plants were independently used by the Iroquois Native American tribe as remedies for diabetes. A compound decoction of any of these plants was taken internally for sugar diabetes.

Yellowspine Thistle (*Cirsium ochrocentrum*). This plant was used by the Zuni Native American tribe as a diabetes remedy. An infusion of the dried or fresh root was taken internally three times, daily for diabetes.

Yellow Bluebeadlily (*Clintonia borealis*). This plant was used by the Iroquois Native American tribe as a diabetes remedy. A compound decoction of the crushed whole plant was taken internally for sugar diabetes.

Pink lady's slipper (Cypripedium acaule).
Lesser yellow lady's slipper (*Cypripedium parviflorum*).
The Cherokee Native American tribe also used these two plant as remedies against diabetes. An infusion of any of these plants was independently taken internally to treat diabetes. A hot infusion of the root could also be taken for the flu.

Queen Anne's lace (*Daucus carota*). This plant was used as a diabetes remedy by the Delaware and Mohegan Native American tribe. An infusion of the fresh flower blossoms (must be in full bloom) was used for diabetes.

Spurge (*Euphorbia sp.*). This plant was used by the Algonquin, Quebec Native American tribe as a diabetes remedy. An infusion of the leaves of this plant was taken for sugar diabetes.

Rocky Mountain Juniper (*Juniperus scopulorum*). The Kutenai Native American tribe used this plant as a diabetes remedy. An infusion was taken internally for sugar diabetes.

Oregon Bitterroot (*Lewisia rediviva*). The Okanagan-Colville Native American tribe used this plant a remedy against diabetes. The fresh or dried roots were eaten to treat diabetes.

Devilsclub (*Oplopanax horridus*). This plant was used by the Gitksan, the Wet'suwet'en and the

Haisla Native American tribes as a diabetes remedy. The bark and other plants were mixed and used for diabetes. The Thompson Native American tribe also took this plant as a diabetes remedy but they took only an infusion of the roots to treat diabetes.

Nightblooming Cereus (*Peniocereus greggii*). This plant was used by the Pima Native American tribes as a remedy for diabetes. A decoction of roots taken to treat diabetes.

Common Selfheal (*Prunella vulgaris*) the Iroquois Native American tribe used this plant as a remedy for sugar diabetes.

Sumac (*Rhus sp.*). The Iroquois used this plant as an emetic. A decoction of the plant's berries was taken as an emetic to treat sugar diabetes. The same plant and application was also used for measles.

Evergreen Huckleberry (*Vaccinium ovatum*). The Pomo, Kashaya Native Indian tribe used this plant as a diabetes remedy. A decoction of the leaves was taken to treat diabetes.

Frost Grape (*Vitis vulpine*). This plant was used by the Chippewa Native American tribe as a remedy for diabetes. An infusion of the plant's root was taken for diabetes.

Adam's Needle (*Yucca filamentosa*). The Cherokee Native American tribe took an infusion of this plant for diabetes remedy.

Sage (*Salvia officinalis*). The Navajo used this plant as a remedy for diabetes. But note that sage has been found to be toxic when taken for the long-term or when taken in excess.

Brazilian Orchid Tree (*Bauhinia forficate*). This tree has been a popular treatment for diabetes because it has the properties to reduce blood sugar levels. Much hypoglycemic activity has been found in the leaves of this plant. An infusion is drunk to treat diabetes, high levels of sugar in the blood, to reduce blood cholesterol levels, urinary and kidney disorders and as a general blood purifier and tonic.

Pfaffia (*Hebanthe eriantha*) or (*Pfaffia paniculata*) This herb is used as general cure-all herbal remedy. It is also used to balance blood sugar levels and to enhance the immune system. Pfaffia is known as a treatment for diabetes, hormonal disorders and imbalances, cancer, high blood pressure, etc. The saponins residing in the roots of Pfaffia include a group of phytochemicals called pfaffosides. These pfaffosides are able to help regulate blood sugar levels.

Prevention of diabetes. While type 1 diabetes is not preventable, type 2 diabetes can be prevented. This can be done by engaging in the following lifestyle changes: eat a healthy diet of fruits, vegetables, whole grains, and lean proteins; exercise moderately for at least 30 minutes, five days per week; maintain a healthy weight; check your blood sugar regularly.

Influenza and Pneumonia

Influenza and Pneumonia are the seventh leading disease cause of mortality in the United States. In 2017, for example, the total number of influenza-and-pneumonia deaths in the United States was 55,672 representing 2% of the total deaths in the United States in 2017.

Influenza (the flu) is a very contagious infection of the influenza virus. There are four major types of the flu virus: (influenza virus Types A, B, C and D). Three of these viruses (Types A, B and C) affect humans, while the fourth virus (Type D) has not affected humans to date. The flu viruses are among the viruses that cause pneumonia.

Pneumonia is an inflammation of the lungs that basically affects the alveoli (the small air sacs in the lungs). Pneumonia causes the alveoli to fill up with fluids thus obstructing oxygen from travelling to the bloodstream. And without enough oxygen in the blood, the body's cells will not function properly or will eventually cease to function at all, causing death. Symptoms of pneumonia typically include fever, chest pain, a mix of both dry and productive cough, and breathing difficulties.

Now let's review some of the anti-influenza/pneumonia herbs and remedies from Native American herbology.

Wild Sarsaparilla (*Aralia nudicaulis*). The Cree Woodlands Native American tribe used this plant as a pediatric aid and as a pulmonary remedy. A decoction of the plant (minus the fruit) was used to treat childhood pneumonia.

Big Sagebrush (*Artemisia tridentate*). The Paiute Native American tribe used this plant as pulmonary aid. A compound decoction of the plant's leaves was taken and a poultice of decoction used for pneumonia. The Shoshoni also used the same plant as a cough medicine and pulmonary aid. The Shoshoni took a decoction of the plant's leaves along with salt to treat both pneumonia and coughs.

Summer Coralroot (*Corallorrhiza maculate*). The Paiute and the Shoshoni Native American tribe used this plant as a blood medicine and as a pulmonary aid. They used the stalks (including an infusion of the dried stalks) of the plant to "build up" pneumonia patients' blood. On the other hand, the Shoshoni

Curlycup Gumweed (*Grindelia squarrosa*). The Crow Native American tribe used this plant as a pulmonary aid. It was given to treat pneumonia and whooping cough. The Paiute used this same plant also as a pulmonary aid. A hot decoction of this plant's young shoots are taken for pneumonia.

Common Hop (*Humulus lupulus*). The Shinnecock Native American tribe used the common hop as a pulmonary aid. They heated a poultice of dried hops in a cloth bag and applied it as a treatment for pneumonia. The Shinnecock also used this plant as a sedative. They used it to make what was described as "nerve medicine".

Western Juniper (*Juniperus occidentalis*). The Paiute also used this plant as a pulmonary aid. A compound decoction of the twigs of this plant was taken for pneumonia, influenza and fever.

Rocky Mountain Juniper (*Juniperus scopulorum*). This plant was used by the Cheyenne, the Nez Perce, the Sioux and the Flathead Native American tribes as a pulmonary aid. An infusion of branches, boughs and cones of the plant was used for pneumonia.

Juniper Wood (*Juniperus sp.*). The Apache Native American tribe used this plant as a pulmonary aid. A poultice the wrapped branches are heated and applied to the back of the pneumonia patient.

Carrotleaf Biscuitroot (*Lomatium dissectum*). The Paiute used this plant as a pulmonary aid and a respiratory aid, in several ways to treat pneumonia. A decoction of dried root was often taken for pneumonia, hay fever and bronchitis. The Shoshoni and the Washo also took this plant as a pulmonary aid. They took a decoction of the root for pneumonia.

Western Sweetroot (*Osmorhiza occidentalis*). This plant was used by the Paiute and the Washo as a pulmonary aid. A decoction of root of the plant was taken for pulmonary disorders including pneumonia. The Shoshoni also used this plant to treat whooping cough. The Shoshoni also sometimes infused the roots of this plant with Indian balsam and took the infusion for pneumonia.

Common Yarrow (*Achillea millefolium*). This plant was used by the Miwok Native American tribe as an analgesic and as a remedy for influenza. The dried or fresh leaves are used during an influenza epidemic and for pain. An Infusion of the flowers and leaves was also used externally for influenza. The Thompson Native American tribe also took an infusion of the flowers of this plant (in small quantities) to treat influenza.

Foothill Sagewort (*Artemisia ludoviciana*). The Paiute used this plant as a disinfectant, an herbal steam and a remedy against influenza. The branches of this plant were used as a bed in a type of sweat-bath to steam out the influenza virus/sickness. The Shoshoni also took a decoction of the branches of this plant as a remedy against influenza.

Butterfly Milkweed (*Asclepias tuberosa*).
Tasselflower Brickellbush (*Brickellia grandiflora*).
Fendler's Bedstraw (*Galium fendleri*).
Common Hop (*Humulus lupulus*).
Oceanspray (*Holodiscus discolor*).
Horehound (*Marrubium vulgare*).
Sharpleaf Valerian (*Valeriana acutiloba*)
The Navajo Native American tribe used all these plants independently and in various ways as remedies against influenza.

Nevada Smokebush (*Psorothamnus polydenius*). The Paiute and the Shoshoni Native American tribes took a decoction of stems of this plant as a remedy for influenza.

Hairy Horsebrush (*Tetradymia comosa*). The Pauite also used this plant as a remedy against influenza. A compound decoction of the stems of the plant was taken for influenza.

Lodgepole Pine (*Pinus contorta*). The Thompson Native Americans used this plant as a remedy against influenza. An infusion of twigs (with needles attached) was prepared and taken for influenza.

Bud Sagebrush (*Picrothamnus desertorum*). The Shoshoni took a decoction of the whole of this plant, also used it as a wash for influenza.

Kidney Disease

Kidney disease is the eighth leading disease cause of mortality in the United States. In 2017, for example, the total number of kidney disease deaths in the United States was 50,046 representing 1.8% of the total deaths in the United States in 2017. Kidney disease refers to three main conditions: nephritis, nephrosis and nephrotic syndrome. Nephritis refers to inflammation of the kidney which can result from an autoimmune disorder, a medication you're taking or an infection. Nephrosis is a kind of kidney disease often resulting from chemical or physical changes that damage the kidneys and which, if not properly treated, may eventually lead to kidney failure. Nephrotic syndrome (another result of kidney damage) is a condition of the kidneys that causes them to produce excess protein in the urine.

And with regard to kidney diseases, Native American herbology also has so many healing secrets, herbs and herbal remedies to offer to humanity. Let's take a look.

Balsam Fir (*Abies balsamea*). The Anticosti Native American tribe used this plant as a kidney aid. They took a decoction of the bark of this plant mixed with the bark of another plant, for kidney troubles. They also ate the gum from this plant for kidney pains. The Iroquois also used this same plant for cancer treatment. They made a poultice of the gum of this plant mixed with dried beaver kidneys and applied it for cancer treatment.

Striped Maple (*Acer pensylvanicum*). This plant was used by the Micmac, Native American tribe, as a kidney aid. The wood was used for kidney problems. The Penobscot tribe also used this plant as a kidney aid. A compound infusion of the plant was taken for kidney problems.

Common Yarrow (*Achillea millefolium*). The Delaware and the Mohegan used this plant as a kidney aid. The Delaware took an infusion of the plant for kidney disorders. And the Mohegan took a compound or simple infusion of leaves of this plant for kidney disorders. The Oklahoma tribe also used this plant as a kidney aid. They took an infusion of the whole plant to treat kidney issues.

Western Yarrow (*Achillea millefolium var. occidentalis*). As for the Paiute, they used as a kidney aid, the Western Yarrow which is a variant of the Common Yarrow. The Paiute took a decoction of the roots of the Western Yarrow to treat kidney troubles.

Black Bugbane (*Actaea racemose*). The Micmac and the Penobscot Native American tribes both used this plant as a kidney aid. They both used the roots of this plant to treat kidney disease.

Indianhemp (*Apocynum cannabinum*). The Cherokee and the Meskwaki Native American tribes both used this plant as a kidney aid. Both tribes used the root of this plant (including as an infusion) to treat kidney problems, dropsy (water accumulation in a part of the body), ague (fever with chills and sweating) and Bright's disease (which today would be called nephritis or glomerulonephritis).

Drummond's Rockcress (*Arabis drummondii*). The Okanagon and the Thompson Native American tribes used this plant as a kidney aid and a urinary aid. The Okanagon took a decoction of the whole plant to treat kidney troubles, while the Thompson also took a decoction of the whole plant to treat kidney troubles and as bladder medicine.

Kinnikinnick (*Arctostaphylos uva-ursi*). This plant was used by the Cherokee Native American tribe as a kidney aid to treat dropsy. The Okanagan-Colville also used it as a kidney aid. A decoction of stems and leaves of the plant was taken as a tonic for the kidneys and the bladder. The Thompson tribe also used the same plant as a tonic. A decoction of stems and leaves was also taken as a tonic for the bladder and the kidneys.

Milkweed (*Asclepias sp.*). The Natchez Native American tribe used this plant as a kidney aid. Members of the tribe took an infusion of the root of this plant for Bright's disease (which today would be called nephritis or glomerulonephritis), nephritis and kidney trouble.

Pipsissewa (*Chimaphila umbellate*). The Kutenai Native American tribe used this plant as a kidney aid. An infusion of the plant was used for kidney trouble. The Micmac also used this herb to treat kidney pain and nondescript kidney troubles. The Okanagan-Colville equally used an infusion of leaves and roots of this plant to "clean out" the kidneys. The Iroquois also used the plant as a kidney aid, using a compound decoction of the roots of the plant to treat dropsy and kidney problems. The Yurok also used the leaves of this plant to treat kidney ailments.

Watermelon (*Citrullus lanatus*). The Cherokee and the Rappahannock Native American tribes used the watermelon as a kidney aid. The Cherokee took an infusion of watermelon seeds to treat kidney trouble. The Rappahannock also took an infusion of watermelon seeds for gravel (kidney stones).

Devil's Darning Needles (*Clematis virginiana*). The Iroquois and the Cherokee used this plant as a kidney aid. An infusion was taken by the Cherokee for the kidneys, while the Iroquois used the plant to treat "burning" kidney troubles.

Squash (*Cucurbita sp.*). The Cheyenne Native American tribe used squash as a kidney aid. They took an infusion of rind for kidney troubles.

Prevention of kidney disease. To prevent kidney disease, you will also need to make the following lifestyle changes: eat a low-sodium diet; quit alcohol and tobacco smoking; exercise moderately for at least 30 minutes daily, five days per week; maintain a healthy weight; get urine and blood tests done regularly (if you have a family history of kidney diseases).

Septicemia

Septicemia is the ninth leading disease cause of mortality in the United States. In 2017, for example, the total number of septicemia deaths in the United States was 38,940 representing 1.42% of the total deaths in the United States in 2017. Septicemia (also known as "blood poisoning") results from a bacterial infection in the blood. Septicemia usually develops from a severe case of infection in a different part of the body (e.g. skin, lungs). Different kinds of bacteria can cause septicemia. The commonest type of infections that can result in septicemia include: infections located around the abdominal area, urinary tract infections, kidney infections and lung infections. When these types of infections become severe, bacteria from the infections can infiltrate the bloodstream and multiply quickly causing septicemia. Septicemia is more common among children, the elderly (75 years old or older), people with immune impairment issues and people suffering chronic illnesses.

Now, here are some Native American herbal/natural solutions for blood poisoning:

Annual Ragweed (*Ambrosia artemisiifolia*). This plant is also known as common ragweed, Roman wormwood, short ragweed, low ragweed or small ragweed. The Delaware Native American tribe used this plant as a blood medicine. They used this plant as a poultice to counteract blood poisoning. The Oklahoma also applied a poultice of this plant to prevent blood poison.

American Spikenard (*Aralia racemose*). The Menominee used this plat as a blood medicine. The root of this plat was used to treat cases of blood poisoning. A poultice of the roots was also used to treat sores.

Tilesius' Wormwood (*Artemisia tilesii*). The Upper Tanana, native American tribe used this plant as a blood medicine. The leaves of this plant were made into a poultice and applied for blood poisoning or a decoction of the leaves of the plant was used as a wash for blood poisoning.

Sacred Thornapple (*Datura wrightii Regel*). The Paiute also used this plant as a blood medicine. The roots were ground and made into a decoction and taken internally in the cases of blood poisoning in the foot.

Redroot Buckwheat (*Eriogonum racemosum*). The Ramah Navajo drank a cold infusion of this whole plant to treat blood poisoning and internal injuries.

Idaho Hymenopappus (*Hymenopappus filifolius*). The Navajo used this plant as a blood medicine. The took a decoction of whole plant for cases of blood poisoning.

Harlequin Blueflag (*Iris versicolor*). The Iroquois used the harlequin blueflag as a blood medicine. The rhizomes were crushed and made into a poultice and used for cases of blood poisoning brought about by contusions.

American Skunkcabbage (*Lysichiton americanus*). The Gitksan Indians used a compound or simple poultice of the pulverized root of this plant and applied it for blood poisoning and boils.

Starry False Solomon's Seal (*Maianthemum stellatum*). The Washo Native American tribe used an infusion of the root of this plant as an antiseptic wash to treat blood poisoning cases.

White Spruce (*Picea glauca*). The Cree Native American tribe used this plant as a blood medicine. They made a poultice if the gum from this plant, mixed it with lard and applied it in cases of blood poisoning.

Pin Cherry (*Prunus pensylvanica*). The Algonquin Indians also used this plant as a blood medicine. They made an infusion out of the bark and took it for blood poisoning.

Red Oak (*Quercus sp.)* The women of the Atsugewi tribe took a decoction to prevent blood poisoning.

Blue Elderberry (*Sambucus nigra*). The Kawaiisu Indians used this plant as a blood medicine. They made a decoction of the leaves of this plant and used it to wash a limb affected by blood poisoning.

European Red Elderberry (*Sambucus racemose*). The Squaxin used an infusion of the leaves of this plant as a wash on the area of the body affected by blood poisoning.

California False Hellebore (*Veratrum californicum*). The Paiute and the Shoshoni tribes used this plant as a gland medicine. They made a poultice of the root of this plant and applied it for cases of blood poisoning and enlarged throat glands.

Prevention of septicemia. To prevent septicemia, treat all bacterial infections quickly and thoroughly. A quick and complete treatment will prevent any bacterial infection in any part of the body from spreading to the blood.

Chronic liver disease

Chronic liver disease is the tenth leading disease cause of mortality in the United States. In 2017, for example, the total number of liver disease deaths in the United States was 38,170 representing 1.39% of the total deaths in the United States in 2017.

Liver disease is a type of disease of or damage to the liver. And when liver disease is unresolved for a long time it becomes chronic liver disease. There are over ninety-five different types of liver disease. But the common ones among them include: fascioliasis, hepatitis, alcoholic liver disease, fatty liver disease, non-alcoholic fatty liver disease, hereditary-diseases-based liver disease, primary liver cancer, primary biliary cirrhosis, primary sclerosing cholangitis, Budd–Chiari syndrome and cirrhosis, etc.

Liver disease can occur through different mechanisms including DNA damage (occasioned by viral infection, obesity and alcohol abuse); the impact of viral infections (such as hepatitis B and C); and the impact of air pollutants (particularly carbon black and particulate matter). Liver disease is commonest among people who use alcohol excessively, people suffering from viral hepatitis and people with fatty liver disease. Liver disease and cirrhosis both result from liver damage.

Cirrhosis is the replacement of healthy liver tissue by scar tissue, thus disrupting the normal functioning of the liver. Scar tissue can slow down the rate of blood flow through the liver. Eventually this will significantly impede the liver from working the way it should. Cirrhosis is a long-term liver disease and its damage builds up over time. In a worst case scenario cirrhosis may cause the liver to cease working entirely (liver failure). The commonest causes of cirrhosis include: alcohol abuse, hepatitis, non-alcoholic fatty liver disease (linked to metabolic syndrome), autoimmune disorders, blocked or damaged bile ducts, use of certain drugs, some parasite infections and exposure to toxic chemicals, etc.

The Native Americans have used several remedies for liver diseases and cirrhosis. These include the following:

Watercress (*Rorippa nasturtium-aquaticum*). The Mahuna Indians used this plant as a liver aid. The plant was used to treat cases of torpid liver, gallstones and cirrhosis of the liver. The Costanoans also used a decoction of this plant as a liver remedy.

Common Yarrow (*Achillea millefolium*). The Blackfoot, the Delaware and the Oklahoma Native American tribes used this plant as a liver aid. An infusion of the whole plant was taken internally or rubbed on the body to treat liver disorders. The Mohegan tribe also drank a compound or simple infusion of the leaves of this plant for liver problems.

Northern Maidenhair (*Adiantum pedatum*). This plant was used by the Iroquois as a liver aid. A decoction of the crushed roots of this plant was taken to treat the cessation of urine due to gall.

Spreading Dogbane (*Apocynum androsaemifolium*). The Iroquois took a decoction of the root of this plant as liver medicine.

American Spikenard (*Aralia racemosa*). The Iroquois also used this plant as a liver aid A compound infusion of this plant was used to treat liver complaints.

Horseflyweed (*Baptisia tinctoria*). The Iroquois also used this plant as a liver aid. They took an infusion of this plant to concentrate bile.

Common Barberry (Berberis vulgaris). The Shinnecock Indians used the common barberry as a liver aid. They took a decoction of the leaves three times daily for jaundice.

Yellow Birch (Betula alleghaniensis). The Delaware Indians also used the yellow birch as a liver aid. A decoction of the bark of the plant was taken to supposedly regulate bile.

The Cherokee Native American tribe had a plethora of remedies for liver problems including:
Nodding Onion (*Allium cernuum*). Juice taken for liver complaints.
Maidenhair Spleenwort (*Asplenium trichomanes*). Taken for liver complaints.
Sharplobe Hepatica (*Hepatica nobilis*). Infusion taken for the liver.
Dwarf Crested Iris (*Iris cristata*). Infusion taken for liver.
Dwarf Violet Iris (*Iris verna*). Infusion taken for liver.
Virginia Iris (*Iris virginica*). Infusion taken for liver.
Purple Passionflower (*Passiflora incarnate*). Infusion taken for liver.
Summer Grape (*Vitis aestivalis*). Infusion of leaf taken for liver.
Fox Grape (*Vitis labrusca*). Infusion of leaf taken for liver.

Frost Grape (*Vitis vulpine*). Infusion of leaf taken for liver.
Indian Physic (*Porteranthus stipulates*). Compound taken for liver.
Bowman's Root (*Porteranthus trifoliatus*). Compound taken for liver.
Culver's Root (*Veronicastrum virginicum*). Compound taken for inactive liver.
Mockernut Hickory (*Carya alba*). Used for bile.
Shellbark Hickory (*Carya laciniosa*). Used for bile.
Sand Hickory (*Carya pallida*). Used for bile
White Colicroot (*Aletris farinosa*). Taken for jaundice.
Virginia Strawberry (*Fragaria virginiana*). Taken for jaundice.
Virginia Creeper (*Parthenocissus quinquefolia*). Infusion taken for yellow jaundice.
Mountain Sweetpepperbush (*Clethra acuminate*). Decoction of bark scrapings taken for vomiting bile.
Common Persimmon (*Diospyros virginiana*). Cold infusion of bark taken for bile and liver.
Wild Hydrangea (*Hydrangea arborescens*). Infusion of bark given to induce vomiting to 'throw off disordered bile.'
Ashy Hydrangea (*Hydrangea cinerea*). Infusion of bark scrapings taken for vomiting bile.
False Aloe (*Manfreda virginica*). Root chewed for the liver.
Dwarf Ginseng (*Panax trifolius*). Used for the liver.

Prevention of liver disease and cirrhosis. To prevent liver disease and cirrhosis, do not use alcohol excessively. If you currently misusing alcohol, seek treatment and quit. The more prolonged and more excessive your abuse of alcohol, the greater your risk of coming down with liver disease or cirrhosis. In addition, if you have hepatitis, be sure to follow the instructions of your doctor and manage the disease well, in order to prevent unnecessary liver damage.

HIV

HIV is not among the top 10 diseases that cause the death of Americans, but it is a very serious disease hence its inclusion in this list.

Creosote bush (*Larrea tridentata*). Creosote bush was used in traditional Native American medicine to treat several illnesses and diseases including respiratory disorders. But today, modern scientific research has found that one compound isolated from the creosote bush (called NDGA or nordihydroguaiaretic acid) has the capacity (as demonstrated in clinical studies) to inhibit cancerous growth. This NDGA compound has also been found to be beneficial to HIV patients for the treatment of HIV. Creosote Bush should be used with care as it has very serious side effects and should be eaten or used only under the supervision of a doctor. Under the supervision of a licensed doctor, the flower buds of creosote bush are usually pickled in vinegar and eaten. Tea can also be made out of the stem and leaves and drank. The twigs may also be chewed.

Carqueja (*Baccharis genistelloides*). This whole plant is antiviral, analgesic, hypoglycemic, anti-inflammatory, abortifacient, tonic and hepatic, etc.

This whole plant is used medicinally. Carqueja is effective against high blood pressure and diabetes, inflammation, stomach acidity and ulcers, among others. It is also used to treat indigestion, sore throat, tonsillitis, diarrhea, angina, anemia, kidney disorders, urinary inflammation, intestinal worms, leprosy, poor blood circulation, malaria and dropsy, etc. Carqueja's antiviral properties have also been confirmed by scientific findings. It has shown activity against vesicular stomatitis and herpes simplex I even at low dosages. In vitro studies have also shown that Carqueja is inhibitive of the replication of HIV virus in T-cell. And this is mainly because of the presence of a compound, 3,5-dicaffeoylquinic acid, in Carqueja. The compound, 3,5-dicaffeoylquinic acid, is an effective inhibitor of the HIV virus even at very low dosages (e.g. only 1 mcg/ml).

Moreton Bay Chestnut (*Castanospermum austral*). This plant is also known by the following names: black bean or bean tree. Only the seed of this plant might be edible if properly cooked and leeched. Do not eat the fresh raw seed as it contains saponins and is toxic. The seeds have been sliced and soaked in running water for no less than ten days, then roasted and ground into a powder and eaten or stored for later use. Very importantly the seeds of this plant contain compounds called castanospermine that are currently being studied for their HIV inhibitory properties. And the seeds could probably be useful in the treatment of AIDS.

Obesity

Woolly Plantain (*Plantago patagonica*). The Navajo Indians and the Ramah Indians used this plant as a dietary aid. A cold infusion of parts of the plants is ingested to decrease appetite, thus preventing obesity.

Colorado four o'clock (*Mirabilis multiflora*). The Zuni Indians used this plant as a dietary aid, a weight reduction herb. The root was crushed into a powder and then combined with flour to make into a bread that when eaten significantly reduces the appetite, for prevention of obesity.

Snowbrush Ceanothus (*Ceanothus velutinus*). The Thompson Indians used this plant as a dietary aid, a weight reduction herb. A decoction of the plant's branches is taken intermittently to trigger weight loss.

Chamisso's Manfern (*Cibotium chamissoi*). The Hawaiians used this plant as a dietary aid, an herb for weight loss. An infusion of the powdered bark of the plant together with other plants are ingested for weight loss.

Male Fern (*Dryopteris filix-mas*). The Bella Coola Indian tribe used this plant as a dietary, weight-loss aid. Specifically, the rhizomes of the plant are eaten raw to trigger weight loss.

Oregon Crabapple (*Malus fusca*). The Nitinaht tribe used this plant as a dietary aid for weight loss and prevention of obesity. An infusion of the bark of this plant was ingested to trigger weight loss and to treat obesity.

Buckthorn (*Rhamnus cathartica*). The buckthorn bark is used for medicinal purposes against obesity. It has also been used as a laxative or purgative. It has also been used for liver health, hepatitis, rheumatism, headache, allergies, intestinal worms, and skin diseases such as acne, eczema, and psoriasis.

Yerba Mate (*Ilex paraguariensis*). As a medicinal herb, it is utilized for many things, particularly obesity. It has also been used for increasing immunity, purifying the blood, minimizing stress and fighting insomnia. It has also been used as a tonic, diuretic, and as a stimulant to reduce fatigue, curb appetite, treat gastric and digestive problems, lower blood pressure, detoxifying the body, nerve pain, depression, insomnia, fever, obesity and to stimulate the nervous and muscular systems.

Stevia (*Stevia rebaudiana*). This plant is also, commonly known as Sugarleaf and Sweetleaf. It is well-known for its use as a sweetener. But it is also used in treating obesity. It has also been used to treat hypertension, diabetes, flatulence and heartburn.

CHAPTER 4: SPECIFIC DISEASES AND CONDITIONS AND THEIR NATIVE AMERICAN HERBAL CURES AND REMEDIES

Asthma

Skunk cabbage (*Symplocarpus foetidus*). Skunk cabbage has been used to treat asthma. This plant was used by the Dakota and Winnebago tribes to trigger the expectoration of phlegm in asthma. The rootstock is also used against nervous disorders, respiratory disorders, dropsy and rheumatism. Skunk cabbage is considered toxic because it has calcium oxalate crystals. However, the toxicity can be eliminated through thorough and precise preparation.

Mullein (*Verbascum thapsus*). The Penobscots, Mohegans and the Forest Potawatomis smoked the dried mullein leaves as treatment for asthma. Dried mullein root was also used for respiratory issues. A sweetened syrup made from the boiled mullein root was used by the Catawba Indians to treat cough in children.

Backache

Horsemint (*Monarda punctata*). This plant is also called "spotted beebalm". The leaves are edible, either cooked or raw and are often used as tea or as flavoring in salads. Many Native American tribes have traditionally taken this plant internally to treat vomiting and nausea. They have also used it externally (in the form of a poultice) to treat rheumatism and swellings. A cold-water infusion of its fresh leaves has been ingested by the Catawba Indian tribe to relieve back pain. Horsemint has also been used to treat fever, chills and inflammation. It can be found in North America from Florida, Louisiana to Long Island, New York.

Arnica (*Arnica montana*). The Catawba applied a hot infusion of Arnica roots to relieve aching backs. Arnica is good for injured muscles, muscle aches, soreness and inflammation and joint swelling and pain, etc. Arnica should never be ingested orally. In fact, Arnica is rarely used in internal medicine as ingestion of undiluted arnica can cause death. Arnica should be applied topically (on the skin) only and never be put in the mouth.

Bronchitis

Creosote bush (Larrea tridentata). Creosote bush is indigenous to the Mojave, Sonoran and Chihuahuan Deserts. It typically lives up to hundreds of years' years. Creosote bush tea is used to treat respiratory ailments such as influenza, cold, cough, tuberculosis, sinusitis and bronchitis. Creosote bush possesses analgesic, anti-inflammatory and antidiarrheal properties. It is also a natural expectorant and helps to expel excess mucus. Today, creosote bush is used to lower cholesterol, to treat cancer, treat HIV and in the multiple treatments of cardiovascular diseases and neurological disorders. Creosote Bush is clearly a super herb, but it has very serious side effects and should only be used under the supervision of a doctor.

Pleurisy root (*Asclepias tuberosa*). CAUTION: this plant is toxic if eaten in large doses, can cause vomiting and diarrhea. Natchez Indians made a tea out of pleurisy root and drank same as a remedy for pneumonia and for the promotion of the expectoration of excess phlegm.

Wormwood (*Artemisia absinthium*). CAUTION: this plant is toxic if used in large doses. Even smaller doses have been known to trigger headaches, convulsions, nervous disorders and insomnia, etc. Avoid if pregnant or breastfeeding or prone to seizures. Nevertheless, Yokia Indians made a tea out of the boiled leaves of wormwood and drank it to treat bronchitis.

Burns

Yellow-spined thistle (*Cirsium ochrocentrum*). Kiowa Indians boiled yellow-spined thistle blossoms and put the tea on skin sores and burns.

Childbirth (for a quick delivery)

Partridgeberry (*Mitchella repens*). During the few weeks leading up to delivery, Cherokee women would boil partridgeberry leaves to make tea and drink until the day of delivery, for easy and quick delivery.

Wild black cherry (*Prunus serotina*). CAUTION: The leaves and seeds of this plant are poisonous!

Handle with care. Cherokee women also made and drank tea made with the inner bark of the wild black cherry herb to reduce pain and discomfort in the early stages of pregnancy.

Broom snakeweed (*Gutierrezia sarothrae*). To help with the ejection of the placenta and to prevent post-partum hemorrhage, Navajo women would make and drink, tea of the whole broom snakeweed plant.

Blue cohosh (*Caulophyllum thalictroides*). This plant is also called "papoose root".   Native Americans have long used the root in tonics, teas and infusions to treat uterine problems and female reproductive issues, to induce labor and to relieve the pains of childbirth.

Black chokecherry (*Prunus virginiana*). Arikara women drank black western chokeberry juice to prevent excessive bleeding.

Buckwheat (*Fagopyrum esculentum*). Hopi women drank a brew of the whole buckwheat plant to halt bleeding.

Smooth sumac (*Rhus glabra*). Omaha women used a hot infusion of smooth sumac fruits as an external wash to relieve the pain of childbirth and to arrest bleeding.

Cotton (*Gossypium hirsutum*). Alabama and Koasati women dank an infusion/tea made from the roots of this plant to reduce labor pains.

Gopher Apple (*Licania michauxii*). The Seminole Indians used the leaves and roots of this plant to ease labor pains and quicken the birth.

Colds

Ginger (*Zingiber officinale*). Ginger was used to deactivate cold viruses and to reduce any accompanying fever.

Licorice (Glycyrrhiza glabra). Licorice was used for congestion relief and for unclogging and freeing the lungs. Licorice also helps to fight off viruses.

Garlic (*Allium sativum*). Garlic was used to halt virus activity. But remember that garlic is more potent when eaten raw (up to 2 cloves a day). You can also make a garlic tea, by crushing several cloves and steeping them in hot water for 5 to 10 hours.

Colic

Catnip (*Nepeta cataria*). The Mohegans treated infant colic with catnip-leaf tea.

Contraceptives

Antelope Sage (*Eriogonum jamesii*). Navajo women made and drank one cup of boiled antelope sage root during menstruation, to inhibit conception.

Milkweed (*Asclepias syriaca*). Post childbirth, Navajo women also made and drank milkweed tea, prepared with the full milkweed plant). To prevent quick conception.

Ragleaf Bahia (*Amauriopsis dissecta*). For the purpose of contraception, the Navajos also drank a tea made of the roots of the ragleaf bahia. The roots were boiled in water for approximately thirty minutes prior to consumption.

American Mistletoe (*Phoradendron leucarpum*). The Mendocino county Indians drank a tea of American mistletoe leaves. This prevented conception or induced abortion.

Dogbane (*Apocynum cannabinum*) A tea made from the boiled roots of the dogbane plant and drank once per week, was used by many tribes for contraceptive purposes.

Blue cohosh (*Caulophyllum thalictroides*). To promote menstruation and parturition, Chippewa women crushed the roots of the blue cohosh herb into powder and made and drank a decoction of the powdered-blue cohosh root.

Indian Paintbrush (*Castilleja affinis*). Hopi women made tea of the full Indian paintbrush plant and drank the tea to dry out the flow of menstruation.

Stoneseed (*Lithospermum*). Shoshoni women were reported to have drank a cold-water brew of stoneseed roots, daily, for six months in order to achieve permanent sterility.

Coughs

Aspen (*Populus tremuloides*). The Cree Indians drank an infusion made from the inner bark of this tree to treat coughs.

Wild Cherry (*Prunus avium*). The Flambeau Ojibwa drank a bark tea of this tree as treatment for coughs and colds, while other tribes also used the bark to treat diarrhea and lung troubles.

White Pine (*Pinus strobus*). The Abnaki Native American tribe used a decoction of the bark of this plant and another plant to treat coughs. The Algonquin made a poultice of the wetted, inner bark and used it on the chest for strong colds. The Delaware used an infusion made of the twigs to treat pulmonary issues. And the Iroquois drank a compound decoction of this plant to treat coughs, colds and rheumatism.

Sarsaparilla (*Smilax officinalis*). The Penobscots combined the crushed dried roots of sarsaparilla and red flag in a warm infusion and drank it as a remedy to cough.

Diabetes

Wild Carrot (*Daucus carota*). CAUTION: The seeds of this plant can be abortifacient. The root can also trigger uterine contractions. So, *Daucus carota* should be avoided by pregnant women. Nonetheless, the Mohegan drank an infusion of the blossoms of wild carrot (when in full bloom) to treat diabetes. An infusion of the plant has also been used in the treatment of several complaints including bladder and kidney issues, dropsy and digestive disorders.

Devil's Club (*Fatsia horrida*). A hot water infusion or tea of the root bark decreases blood sugar considerably and counteracts the effects of diabetes, without toxic effects.

See also all the entries under "Diabetes", in the chapter, above, on the top leading disease-causes of death in the United States.

Diarrhea

Black cherry (*Prunus serotina*). CAUTION: The leaves and seeds of this plant are poisonous! A tea made of the roots has been used the Indians of northern California to treat diarrhea. The Mohegan also fermented ripe black cherry for about a year, then drank the juice as a cure for dysentery.

Alternateleaf Dogwood (*Cornus alternifolia*) or **Silky Dogwood** (*Cornus amomum*). To treat diarrhea, the Menominee either boiled the inner bark of the alternateleaf dogwood or boiled the bark of the silky dogwood and injected the warm liquid into the rectum with a rectal syringe (crafted from hollow bird bone and mammal bladder).

Geranium (*Geranium*). CAUTION: Using this plant may bring on some side effects including nausea, vomiting and headache. Nonetheless, the Chippewa and the Ottawa drank a warm tea made from the boiled whole plant as treatment for diarrhea.

White Oak (*Quercus alba*). The Iroquois and the Penobscot drank a tea made from the boiled bark of the white oak as treatment for bleeding piles and diarrhea.

Black Raspberry (*Rubus occidentalis*). The Pawnee, the Omaha and the Dakota drank an infusion made from the boiled root bark of black raspberry as treatment for dysentery and other bowel problems.

Star Grass (*Aletris farinose*). Other names for this plant include: colic-root, starwort, ague-root, ague grass, bitter grass, Bettie grass, crow corn, devil's bit and true unicorn root, etc. CAUTION: The rhizome of this plant can be toxic if consumed in excess quantities, causing diarrhea, colic and vomiting. Star grass can be found in eastern North America, particularly in Tennessee, Virginia, and North Carolina. The Catawba drank a cold-water tea/infusion of star grass leaves to treat dysentery, stomach aches. It was also used to treat snakebite, irregular periods, menstrual pain, prolapsed uterus, loss of appetite, flatulence, indigestion, bloating, rheumatism and chronic bronchitis.

Digestive Disorders
Dandelion (*Taraxacum officinale*). The Ojibwa drank a tea made of the root of this plant to treat heartburn. The Mohegan drank a tea of the leaves as a tonic.

Yellowroot (*Xanthorhiza simplicissima*). A tea from the root of this plant has been used by the Cherokee and the Catawba as a remedy for stomach ache.

Fevers

Boneset (*Eupatorium perfoliatum*). The Menominee made and drank tea made of boneset in order to reduce fever. The Iroquois and the Mohegan also made and drank a boneset tea for fever and colds. The Creek Indians also made and drank boneset tea for body pain relief. And the Alabama also made and drank a boneset tea for relief from stomach ache.

Bunchberry Dogwood (*Cornus Canadensis*). The Delaware and the Algonkian Indians boiled the inner bark of this plant in water and drank the tea to reduce fevers and body pains.

Willow (*Cornus sp.*). The Pomo tribe boiled the inner bark of the root of this plant and then drank the tea to induce sweating in cases of fever and chills. The Natchez used the bark of the red willow for their fever remedies, while the Creek and the Alabama Indians took willow-root baths in bathwater infused with willow root, as treatment for fever.

Feverwort (*Triosteum perfoliatum*). The Cherokee drank a decoction of the coarse, leafy herb to treat fevers.

Headache

Common Yarrow (*Achillea millefolium*). The Algonquin used the common yarrow as an analgesic. They took a decoction of the plant's flowers and leaves to treat headaches or crushed the leaves and snuffed it to treat headaches. The Chippewa either steamed a decoction of the leaves and inhaled it as a treatment for headache or they splashed a decoction of the leaves on a hot stone (as herbal steam) and inhaled for headache. The Goshute took an infusion of this plant as an analgesic against headache. The Iroquois also used an infusion of the leaves or roots of this plant (externally or internally) to treat headache. The Mendocino and the Okanagan-Colville used this plant, too, as an analgesic. They took an infusion of the flowers and leaves to treat headaches.

Balsam Fir (*Abies balsamea*). The Chippewa melted the gum of this plant on warm stone and inhaled the fumes as treatment for headache.

Candle Anemone (*Anemone cylindrical*). The Meskwaki took an infusion of the root of this plant for headache and dizziness.

Lesser Burdock (*Arctium minus*). The Abnaki took this plant as an analgesic for headaches.

Big Sagebrush (*Artemisia tridentata*). The Kawaiisu inhaled fumes of a decoction of this plant to treat headaches.

Canadian Mint (*Mentha arvensis*). The Paiute used the Canadian mint as an analgesic. They used the leaves of the plant in various ways to treat headaches.

Golden Zizia (*Zizia aurea*). This plant was used by the Meskwaki as a febrifuge (a fever-reducing compound). The root of the plant was taken for fevers, while a compound made up of the plant's flower stalks was taken for headaches.

Heart and circulatory problems

Green Hellebore (*Helleborus viridis*). CAUTION: All parts of this plant are poisonous and it is possible to absorb this poison through the skin. Use only under the strict supervision of a licensed doctor. This plant has been used for hypertension and to reduce blood pressure. The Cherokee have also used the green hellebore to relieve body pains.

Spreading Dogbane (*Apocynum androsaemifolium*).

Downy Yellow Violet (*Viola pubescens*).

The Potawatomi used these two plants as heart medicines. They took a decoction of the green berries of spreading dogbane to treat heart problems and the root of downy yellow violet was taken for different heart diseases.

See also all the entries under "Heart disease", in the chapter, above, on the top leading disease-causes of death in the United States.

Hemorrhoids

White Oak (*Quercus alba*). The Menominee tribe treated hemorrhoids by making an infusion of the inner bark of white oak and injecting it into the rectum with a rectal syringe (made from a hollow bird bone and the bladder of a mammal).

Herpes zoster (shingles)

St. John's Wort (*Hypericum perforatum*). Shingles (herpes zoster) is an infection of the sensory nerves by the herpes zoster virus. This is the same virus that causes chickenpox. St. John's Wort has been used with success for shingles and nerve pain. This herb eases the pain and duration of the herpes zoster virus. About 900 milligrams of the powdered herb should be taken three to 3 to 4 times daily to treat the herpes zoster virus.

Licorice root (*Glycyrrhiza glabra*) has also been used with success against the herpes zoster virus. The herb has anti-inflammatory and antiviral properties and it has a soothing effect on the affected nerve tissue. Also, about 900 milligrams of the powdered herb should be taken 3 to 4 times daily to treat the herpes zoster virus. Also some herbs may be applied as a poultice, salve or compress on the rash to soothe the itching and pain.

Button Brittlebush (*Encelia frutescens*). The Kayenta, Navajo used this plant as a dermatological aid against shingles.

Calendula (*Calendula officinalis*), **Comfrey** (*Symphytum officinale*), **Chaparral** (*Larrea* *tridentate*), **Arnica** (*Arnica montana*) and, **St. John's wort** (*Hypericum perforatum*) are all effective against shingles.

Indigestion

Lesser Yellow Lady's Slipper (*Cypripedium parviflorum*). Small doses of an infusion of the root was taken for indigestion.

Old Man's Whiskers (*Geum triflorum*). A compound decoction of the root was ingested for indigestion.

Alum Root (*Heuchera sp.*). *A compound decoction of the root was ingested for indigestion.*

Cutleaf Coneflower (*Rudbeckia laciniata*). A compound infusion made from the root of this plant has been taken internally to treat indigestion.

Broadleaf Arrowhead (*Sagittaria latifolia*). An infusion of the root of this plant was taken for indigestion.

Salix sp. A compound decoction of the inner bark of this plant was ingested for indigestion.

Inflammations and swellings

Common Plantain (*Plantago major*). The Chippewa, used a compound or simple poultice of the chopped fresh leaf or root of this plant to treat inflammations. The Iroquois used an infusion of the seeds to lessen intestinal inflammation. The Potawatomi used a poultice of the heated plantain leaf on inflammations and swellings to reduce them. And the Shinnecock applied a poultice made of pounded plantain leaves to reduce inflammation in sore spots.

American Spikenard (*Aralia racemose*). The Potawatomi used this plant as a dermatological aid. They prepared and applied a hot poultice of the pounded root of this plant to inflammations.

Canadian Wildginger (*Asarum canadense*). This plant was used by the Chippewa as a dermatological aid. A compound poultice of the chopped root of this plant was applied on inflammations to treat and reduce the inflammation.

Leatherleaf (*Chamaedaphne calyculata*). This plant was also used by the Potawatomi as a dermatological aid. They made a poultice of the leaves and applied the poultice to the inflamed area to reduce the inflammation.

Sweet Fern (*Comptonia peregrine*). The Micmac used sweet fern as an analgesic. The root was used to treat inflammation and headache.

Southern Bayberry (*Morella cerifera*). The Micmac used the root of this plant as both an anti-rheumatic and a dermatological aid. A hot poultice of the roots was prepared and applied on inflammations to reduce them.

Influenza

Common Yarrow (*Achillea millefolium*). The Miwok and the Thompson used this plant as an analgesic and as a disease remedy. The Miwok used the mashed leaves for pain relief and to treat influenza. They also used an infusion of the flowers and leaves (externally) to treat influenza. The

Thompson used an infusion of the plant's flowers (but in smaller quantities) to also treat influenza.

Foothill Sagewort (*Artemisia ludoviciana*). The Paiute used the branches of this plant as a disinfectant and as an herbal steam (as a bed in a sweat bath) to steam out influenza. The Shoshoni also took a decoction of the branches of this pant as a remedy against influenza.

Nevada Smokebush (*Psorothamnus polydenius*). The Shoshoni also used a decoction of the stems of this plant as another remedy against influenza.

See also all the entries under "Influenza and Pneumonia", in the chapter, above, on the top leading disease-causes of death in the United States.

See also all the entries under the chapter on "Special Native American herbal remedies for making yourself flu-proof".

Insect bites and stings
Fendler Bladderpod (*Lesquerella fendleri*). The Navajos made a tea of this plant and used it to treat spider bites.

Common Maidenhair (*Adiantum capillus-veneris*). The Kayenta Navajo used this plant as a dermatological aid. They used an infusion of this plant used as a lotion for centipede and bumblebee stings.

Sassafras (*Sassafras albidum*). The Koasati made a poultice of the crushed leaves of this plant and applied it to bee stings.

Russet Buffaloberry (*Shepherdia Canadensis*). The Carrier ate the froth, the ripe berries or the jelly from this plant to lessen injury from mosquito bites.

Prickly Russian Thistle (*Salsola tragus*). The Navajo used this plant as a dermatological aid. They made a poultice of the chewed plant and applied it to bee, ant and wasp stings.

Fendler's Globemallow (*Sphaeralcea fendleri*). The Navajo used this plant as a dermatological aid to treat sand cricket bites.

Velvet Mesquite (*Prosopis velutina*). The Papago applied a poultice of the chewed leaves of this plant to red ant stings.

Granite Pricklygilia (*Leptodactylon pungens*). The Navajo used this plant to treat scorpion stings.

Pillar False Gumweed (*Vanclevea stylosa*). The Kayenta Navajo, made a compound poultice of this plant and applied it to solpugid (wind scorpion) bites or tarantula bites.

Chaparral Dodder (*Cuscuta californica*). The Diegueno used this plant as an antidote. An infusion of this plant (picked from buckwheat plants) was ingested to treat bites from the black widow spider.

Sand Gilia (*Gilia leptomeria*). The Kayenta Navajo used this plant as a dermatological aid. A poultice of the plant was applied to worm bites and scorpion stings for

Meadow Garlic (*Allium canadense*). The Mahuna rubbed this plant on the body to prevent scorpion, lizard or tarantula bites.

Virginia Snakeroot (*Aristolochia serpentaria*). The Rappahannock made a compound poultice of the crushed roots of this plant and used it as a salve for spider bites.

Woolly Prairieclover (*Dalea lanata*). The Kayenta Navajo used this drug as a dermatological aid. They applied a poultice of this plant to treat centipede bites.

Sacred Thornapple (*Datura wrightii*). The Mahuna used this plant as an anti-venom to treats tarantula bites.

Inland Saltgrass (*Distichlis spicata*). A decoction of this plant was ingested as treatment for pimple-causing doodle bug bites.

Scabland Penstemon (*Penstemon deustus*). The Paiute made a poultice of the crushed fresh leaves of this plant and applied it to tick bites and mosquito bites.

Jewelweed (*Impatiens capensis*). The fresh juice of this plant was used as a wash to treat poison ivy rash or nettle stings by the Potawatomi Indians.

Great Ragweed (*Ambrosia trifida*). The Cherokee used this plant as a dermatological aid. The leaves were crushed and made into a poultice which was rubbed on insect stings, while an infusion of the leaves was used on hives.

Common Plantain (*Plantago major*). The Cherokee used this plant as an antidote to bit poison. They used an infusion of the plant for poisonous stings, bites and snakebites.

Fremont's Cottonwood (*Populus fremontii*). The Diegueno used this pant as a dermatological aid. They used a poultice of the leaves of this plant and applied it to wounds, bruises or insect stings. Alternatively, they used an infusion of the leaves of this plant as a wash to treat wounds, bruises or insect stings.

Insect repellents, insecticides

Sweet After Death (*Achlys triphylla*). The Saanich used this plant as an insecticide. The dried leaves were hung in houses to drive mosquitos and flies away. The Thompson also used a decoction of this same plant as a floor and furniture wash to eliminate and prevent bedbugs, lice and other household pests.

Tapertip Onion (*Allium acuminatum*).
Nodding Onion (*Allium cernuum*).
The Salish rubbed the bulbs of either of these onion species on their skin to repel insects.

Wormwood (*Artemisia dracunculus*). The Keres used wormwood as an insecticide. They crushed the plant, mixed it with water and sprinkled it on beddings as a bed bug repellent. The Shuswap used wormwood also as an insecticide. They burned the plant to keep mosquitos away.

Mockernut Hickory (*Carya alba*). The Choctaw scattered the leaves of this plant around the home and environment to drive away fleas.

Snowbrush Ceanothus (*Ceanothus velutinus*). The Shuswap used this plant as an insecticide. They burnt the plant and the smoke from the plant killed bedbugs.

Rocky Mountain Juniper (*Juniperus scopulorum*). The Shuswap also used this plant to eliminate bedbugs and earwigs from the house.

California Poppy (*Eschscholzia californica*). The Costanoan rubbed a decoction of the flowers of this plant, into the hair to eliminate lice.

Broom Snakeweed (*Gutierrezia sarothrae*). The Jemez burned this plant in a slow fire and the smoke killed bees.

Black Walnut (*Juglans nigra*). The Delaware scattered the leaves of this plant about the house and their environment to dispel fleas.

California Laurel (*Umbellularia californica*). The Yurok put this plant under the bed to eliminate fleas.

Eastern Redcedar (*Juniperus virginiana*). The Cherokee used this plant to moth-proof their houses.

Indian Tobacco (*Lobelia inflate*). The Cherokee also burnt this plant to smoke out gnats.

Eastern Arborvitae (*Thuja occidentalis*). The Iroquois put branches of this plant in closets to ward off moths.

Mayapple (*Podophyllum peltatum*). The Menominee sprinkled a decoction of the whole plant on potato plants to kill bugs that infest potatoes.

Balsam Poplar (*Populus balsamifera*). The Carrier used the resin from the buds of this plant to ward off black flies, mosquitoes and gadflies.

Field Pansy (*Viola bicolor*).
Marsh Blue Violet (*Viola cucullata*).
Downy Yellow Violet (*Viola pubescens*).
Roundleaf Yellow Violet (*Viola rotundifolia*).
Common Blue Violet (*Viola sororia*).
Birdfoot Violet (*Viola pedata*).
The Cherokee used all the above as insecticides. Before planting, seed corn was soaked inside an infusion of any of the above plants to prevent insects or other bugs from being attracted to or attacking the seed corns after they have been planted.

Rheumatism

Pokeweed (*Phytolacca americana*). Virginia Indians ingested an infusion or tea of crushed, boiled berries of this plant to treat rheumatism. The dried root of this plant was also used to relieve inflammation.

Bloodroot (*Sanguinaria Canadensis*). CAUTION: Bloodroot root is toxic. Consuming it in excessive quantities causes nausea, vomiting and a depression of the central nervous system. In extreme cases, it may be fatal. Avoid using this plant if pregnant or breastfeeding. And use only under the supervision of a licensed doctor. Nevertheless, the Mississippi-region Indians have used bloodroot as an effective remedy for rheumatism. And the Rappahannock of Virginia also ingested an infusion or tea of the root of this plant to treat rheumatism.

Balsam Fir (*Abies balsamea*). The Iroquois took a compound decoction of this plant as a remedy against rheumatism.

White Fir (*Abies concolor*). The Keres used an infusion of the foliage of this tree as a bath to treat rheumatism. They also ingested an infusion made of the foliage of this tree as treatment for rheumatism.

Red Baneberry (*Actaea rubra*). The Okanagon took a decoction of the roots of this plant internally to treat rheumatism. The Thompson also took a decoction of the roots internally to treat rheumatism. And the Iroquois used the plant externally. An infusion of roots was used as an anti-rheumatic wash.

Northern Maidenhair (*Adiantum pedatum*). The Cherokee used this plant as an anti-rheumatic. Externally, they rubbed a decoction of the roots of this plant on the rheumatic area of the body and, internally, they ingested an infusion of this plant also to treat rheumatism. The Iroquois also used a compound decoction of the green roots of this plant, externally, as a foot-soak to treat rheumatism. They also ingested a compound decoction of the green roots of this plant as treatment for rheumatism.

Utah Juniper (*Juniperus osteosperma*). The Paiute used this plant as a dermatological aid. They applied a poultice of the crushed twigs of the plant to treat rheumatism or swellings.

Rocky Mountain Juniper (*Juniperus scopulorum*). The Swinomish used this plant externally as an anti-rheumatic remedy. To treat rheumatism, they soaked their feet in an infusion of the roots of this plant.

Eastern Redcedar (*Juniperus virginiana*). The Chippewa used this plant as an internal anti-rheumatic remedy. They ingested a compound decoction made of the twigs of this plant, as treatment for rheumatism.

Creosotebush (*Larrea tridentate*). The Diegueno used this plant externally as an anti-rheumatic remedy. A decoction of the leaves of this plant was used as a bath for painful arthritis and rheumatism. The Pima used the same plant internally as an anti-rheumatic. They ingested an infusion of this plant to treat rheumatism. The Yavapai also used a decoction of the stems and leaves of the creosote bush as a wash for rheumatism. The Isleta also used a decoction of the plant, externally, as a body wash, against rheumatism. The Paiute used an infusion of the leaves of the creosote bush as a wash to treat rheumatism. And the Papago made a poultice of the heated branches of this plant and applied it on the affected area for rheumatism.

Sedatives

Wild black cherry (*Prunus serotina*). This plant is also known as wild cherry or chokecherry. CAUTION: The leaves and seeds of this plant are poisonous! Handle with care. The bark and the fruit of this plant are edible and are used medicinally. The bark is also used as a mild sedative. The Meskwaki made a sedative tea out of the root bark of this plant.

Common Hop (*Humulus lupulus*). The Shinnecock used the common hop as a sedative. They used it to make what was described as "nerve medicine". The Mohegan also prepared a sedative medicine from the cone-like strobiles.

Wild Lettuce (*Lactuca virosa*). CAUTION: this plant is poisonous, although poisoning cases attributed to this plant have been very rarely recorded. Use this plant only under the direct supervision of a licensed doctor. Nevertheless, this plant has been used for sedative purposes, especially regarding nervous complaints. This plant contains 'lactucarium', a sedative which is not addictive and which has the effects of weak opium. It also contains 'hyoscyamine', a depressant.

Stinking Chamomile (*Anthemis cotula*). This plant is also known as Mayweed. CAUTION. The whole plant may cause allergies in sensitive people. Avoid if pregnant or breastfeeding. The Iroquois used this plant as a sedative. A cold infusion of the dried stems and roots were ingested for their sedative effect. The Cherokee also used this same plant as a sedative to treat hysterics.

Field Sagewort (*Artemisia campestris*). The Lakota used this plant as a sedative. The crushed roots of the plant were put on the face of a sleeping man so that his horse could be easily stolen while he deeply sleeps.

Crinkleroot (*Cardamine diphylla*). The Micmac used the root of this plant as a sedative.

Yerba Buena (Clinopodium douglasii). The Mahuna took an infusion of this plant as a sedative for insomnia.

Button Eryngo (*Eryngium yuccifolium*). The Creek used this plant as a sedative, specifically to produce a feeling of tranquility and peace.

Virginia Strawberry (*Fagaria virginiana*). The Cherokee took an infusion of this plant to calm the nerves.

Showy Frasera (*Frasera speciose*). The Navajo used this plant as a sedative to treat nervousness and alarm.

Skin conditions

Subalpine Fir (*Abies lasiocarpa*). The Flathead pounded the needles of this plant and used it mixed with marrow or grease to treat skin diseases or they used the pounded needles alone to treat skin diseases.

Common Yarrow (*Achillea millefolium*). The Chippewa made a decoction of the roots of this plant and applied it to treat skin eruptions. The Kutenai also used a decoction of this plant to wash sores and skin problems. The Paiute made a decoction of the stems and leaves of this plant and used it as a liniment to treat sores and skin issues, while the Thompson made a poultice of the pounded roots of this plant and used it on the skin to treat sciatica. The Thompson also either made an infusion of this plant and used it as wash or they powdered the leaf and the stem of this plant and applied it to the skin to treat skin problems.

White Alder (*Alnus rhombifolia*). The Pomo used a decoction of the bark of this tree as a wash for babies with skin disease. They also used a decoction of the bark as a wash for skin diseases such as diaper rash, sores, itching or peeling skin.

Maile (*Alyxia oliviformis*). The Hawaiian made an infusion of the pounded plant along with other plants and used same in a sweat bath to treat cases of yellow blotches on the skin.

Prairie Broomweed (*Amphiachyris dracunculoides*). The Comanche made a poultice of the boiled flowers of this plant and used it for skin rashes and eczema.

Annual Ragweed (*Ambrosia artemisiifolia*). The Mahuna used an infusion of this plant as a wash for scalp diseases and minor skin eruptions.

California Nettle (*Urtica dioica*). The Tolowa made a poultice of the crushed fresh leaves of this plant which they applied to the skin for skin inflammations.

Common Mullein (*Verbascum Thapsus*). The Zuni made a poultice of powdered root of this plant and applied it to rashes, sores and skin infections.

Adam's Needle (*Yucca filamentosa*). The Catawba took a decoction of the roots of this plant or rubbed the rots on the body to treat skin disease.

Small Soapweed (*Yucca glauca*). The Cheyenne applied the powdered roots of this plant as powder or used it with water as a wash for scabs, sores and skin outbreaks. The Kiowa used the plant to treat baldness, dandruff and skin irritations.

Post Oak (*Quercus stellate*). The Cherokee applied an infusion of the bark of this tree to sores and chapped skin.

Smooth Sumac (*Rhus glabra*). The Nez Perce used this plant as a dermatological aid. The leaves were moistened and applied to the skin for skin rashes. The Omaha made a poultice of the fruits or leaves of this same plant and applied it to the skin in cases of poisoning of the skin. The Sioux also made a poultice of the wetted and powdered fruits or leaves of this plant and also used it for poisoned skin.

Rubber Rabbitbrush (*Ericameria nauseosa*). The Klamath made a poultice of the smashed plant and applied it to blisters or used it to raise blisters.

Turkish Rugging (*Chorizanthe staticoides*). The Tubatulabal used an infusion of the whole Turkish rugging plant as a lotion for pimples.

Greene's Rabbitbrush (*Chrysothamnus greenei*). The Navajo made an infusion of the tops of this plant and used it as a wash for measles and chickenpox eruptions.

Chicory (*Cichorium intybus*). The Iroquois used a decoction of the roots of this plant as a wash for fever sores and chancres or they made a poultice of this plant and applied it to fever sores and chancres for relief.

Field Thistle (*Cirsium discolor*). The Iroquois either took a compound decoction of the roots of this plant or made and applied a poultice of the roots of this plant to treat boils.

Rock Clematis (*Clematis Columbiana*). The Okanagan-Colville made an infusion of the leaves or an infusion of the leaves and stems and used it as a hair wash to prevent the appearance of gray hair. The Okanagan-Colville also made a poultice of the wetted and pounded leaves of this plant and applied it to the feet, to treat sweaty feet.

Western White Clematis (*Clematis ligusticifolia*). The Thompson also used this plant as a dermatological aid. They used the plant as a head wash and for eczema and scabs.

Thrush

Atlantic Pigeonwings (*Clitoria mariana*). The Cherokee prepared and held an infusion of this plant in the mouth for 10 to 20 minutes to treat thrush.

Common Persimmon (*Diospyros virginiana*). The Catawba boiled the tree bark in water and the resulting dark liquid was used as a mouth rinse for thrush. The Cherokee also made a syrup of this plant and used it to treat thrush.

Spotted Geranium (*Geranium maculatum*). The Cherokee used a compound decoction of this plant as a pediatric mouth wash for infant thrush. They also used a decoction of this plant mixed with fox grapes as a pediatric mouth wash for infant thrush.

Bigseed Biscuitroot (*Lomatium macrocarpum*). The Okanagan-Colville made a poultice of the pounded roots of this plant and applied it to the inside of babies mouths to treat thrush and mouth sores.

American Ginseng (*Panax quinquefolius*). The Cherokee also used an infusion of this plant to treat thrush.

Resurrection Fern (*Pleopeltis polypodioides*). The Houma made a cold decoction of the fronds of this plant and used it as a wash for babies' thrush and sore mouths.

Summer Grape (*Vitis aestivalis*). The Cherokee used a compound decoction of this plant to wash a child's mouth as treatment for thrush.

Fox Grape (*Vitis labrusca*). The Cherokee also used a compound decoction of this plant to wash a child's mouth as treatment for thrush.

Frost Grape (*Vitis vulpine*). The Cherokee also used a compound decoction of this plant to wash a child's mouth as treatment for thrush.

Tilesius' Wormwood (*Artemisia tilesii*). The Tanana made a decoction of the above-ground parts of this plant and ingested it as treatment for mouth sores.

Yeast infections
Prairiesmoke (*Geum triflorum*). The Okanagan-Colville women took an infusion of the roots of this plant to treat vaginal yeast infection.

California Sagebrush (*Artemisia californica*). The Mahuna women took infusion of this plant to treat "vaginal troubles".

CHAPTER 5: THE MOST-IMPORTANT HERBS THAT NATIVE AMERICANS USED EVERYDAY TO CURE EVERYTHING

Native Americans are noted for their vast knowledge of herbs and medicinal plants. They have been masters of their environment who knew what was available to them in their environment, how to find these resources and how to use those resources for their own benefit. It is believed that Native Americans first got the idea of putting plants and herbs to therapeutic use by observing how some sick animals tended to seek out and eat certain plants whenever they were sick. From there, more and more herbal/medicinal plant knowledge was acquired and preserved through ages of trial and error and oral tradition, cumulating to the vast expanse of knowledge of effective natural therapies that Native Americans have bequeathed to the world today.

Here are some of the most resourceful plants that the Native Americans used in their everyday lives and the knowledge of which they have bequeathed to us today. All of these plants are still in therapeutic use today and all are still effective and complementary to modern medicine. Many of them are today used as alternative treatments and are considered to be, arguably, more effective, natural, safer and more holistic than modern pharmaceutical solutions. Let us review some of these versatile herbs:

Ashwagandha. (*Withania somnifera*). This plant is also called winter cherry, Indian ginseng or poison gooseberry. CAUTION: This plant is toxic if eaten. Do not use in pregnancy or breastfeeding, as the whole plant (but particularly the root, bark and leaves) are abortifacient, narcotic and strongly sedative. Nevertheless, Native Americans used ashwagandha as a sedative and to treat memory loss, rheumatism, muscle tension/weakness, bone weakness and loose teeth. It has also been used as a tonic for revitalizing and rejuvenating the body and is particularly helpful with recovery after sickness. The bark, root and leaves of this plant contain antibiotic properties. And a poultice has been made out of this plant and used to treat pains and all kinds of swelling. Ashwagandha has also been used as a tranquillizer.

It has also been taken internally to restore post-miscarriage normalcy to the uterus, to treat post-partum problems, debility, nervous exhaustion, wasting disease, insomnia, impotence, multiple sclerosis and failure to stunted thriving in children, etc. Externally it has been applied as a poultice to boils, swellings and other external points of pain in the body.

Blackberry (*Rubus allegheniensis*). This plant is also known as the common blackberry. This plant is very common in central and eastern North America. It is native to some locations in California and

British Columbia. Recent studies have found that blackberries are rich in essential compounds, antioxidants, and bioflavonoids. Native Americans have used blackberries to treat stomach disorders. The roots have been confirmed to have anti-inflammatory ingredients that are effective for treating joint pains and reducing all forms of swelling. The roots have also been blended, sweetened with honey and used to treat mouth sores, sore throat, bleeding gums and cough.

Black gum bark (*Nyssa sylvatica*). The Cherokee often used the twigs and the bark of this tree to make tea to ease chest pains. The twigs were also used for cleaning the teeth.

Buckbrush (*Ceanothus cuneatus*). This plant is also known as *redstem ceanoathus*, hummingbird blossom, mountain lilac, Oregon teatree, Jersey tea and snowbush. Buckbrush roots have been used by Cherokee medicinal healers since the roots have diuretic properties that are capable of stimulating the kidney. Other parts of this plant have also been found effective for treating throat and mouth infections, tumors, cysts, inflammation, swollen spleens and lymph nodes, hemorrhoids and inflamed tonsils. The plant has also been used for post-natal care. The roots and bark of this plant as used medicinally mostly in the form of a tea. To prepare the tea, boil water and dip the backbrush barks and roots inside the water for about five minutes and drink while warm.

Cattail (*Typha latifolia*). This plant is also called reedmace, broad-leaved cattail, cat-o'-nine-tails, bulrush, common cattail, common bulrush, candlewick, cooper's reed, great reedmace, corn dog grass or cumbungi. CAUTION: Do not use while pregnant or breastfeeding. This plant absorbs pollutants and, in fact, has been used as a bioremediator, so do not eat any harvest of this plant that derives from polluted water. Also do not eat if the harvest tastes very spicy or very bitter. Cattail is native to all states in the United States (with the exception of Hawaii). And in Canada, it can be found in every province, including the Yukon and the Northwest Territories. Native Americans have primarily used this plant as a means of healthful sustenance during the recovery process from sickness.

This plant is also named the "supermarket of the swamp" and this is because of its versatility as it is eaten in several different ways. The young shoots of this plant can be eaten cooked or raw and have been eaten to treat diarrhea. The immature, green spikes can also be cooked and eaten. The yellow pollen of this plant can be collected and mixed with other flours to create a protein-rich flour mixture. The sprouts can be eaten cooked or raw. The sprouts' starchy core be cooked like potato. And the starchy root stocks can be dried cooked and eaten like potato or milled into flour to be eaten.

In terms of medicinal use, the leaves of this plant are diuretic. They have been combined with oil into a poultice and used on sores. The dried pollen is used internally to treat hemorrhage, painful menstruation, kidney stones, post-partum pains, abscesses, abnormal bleeding from the uterus and lymphatic system cancer. This plant is also used to treat diarrhea, tapeworms and injuries. A decoction made of the stems has also been used to treat whooping cough. The roots have been crushed and used as a poultice and applied on cuts, wounds, sores, boils, inflammations, carbuncles, scalds and burns. The flowers of this plant have also been used to treat a variety of disorders including amenorrhea, abdominal pain, dysuria, cystitis, vaginitis and metrorrhagia.

Curly dock (*Rumex crispus*). This herb is also known as yellow dock, curled dock, narrow dock, sour dock or rumex. CAUTION: curly dock may aggravate arthritis, rheumatism, kidney stones, gout or hyperacidity. And since the leaves contain high levels of oxalic acid, the leaves should not be consumed in large quantities. Cooking will, however, reduce the oxalic acid content. Nevertheless, the herb is a familiar ingredient in salads. The leaves and stems can be eaten cooked or raw or dried and stored for later use. The leaves can be added to salads, soups or prepared as a potherb. The seeds can also be eaten cooked or raw. They can also be ground into powder and used as flour or roasted and consumed as a substitute for coffee. They have also been used to treat diarrhea. This herb is rich in health-promoting minerals and vitamins (especially vitamins A, C and iron) and its taste is a combination of sweetness and sourness. Native Americans used it as a laxative and a tonic. The plant can be blended to powder, mixed with beeswax and oil and applied as an ointment to relieve skin irritations, cuts, sores and rashes.

Also, the herb has good cleansing properties and is used to treat different skin problems. All parts of this plant can be put to medicinal use, but the root is the most potent, medicinally. Depending on the dose taken, it can trigger or alleviate diarrhea. It is taken internally to treat diarrhea, constipation, bleeding of the lungs, piles, a wide range of blood complaints and chronic skin diseases. The root is mashed and used externally as a poultice or salve or dried and used as dressing powder on ulcers, wounds, sores and other skin problems. The root has also been used effectively against cancer.

Devil's claw (*Harpagophytum procumbens*). While the name may to portray this plant as dangerous, Native Americans have employed it for the treatment of various health conditions such as fever, digestion issues, arthritis and skin diseases. An infusion/tea of this plant works to reduce diabetes. A decoction made from the roots is used to treat sores, joint pain, back pain, arthritis, headache, gout and to lessen swelling.

Geranium. (*Geranium*). Geranium is a genus of about 422 species that are known as geraniums, also as cranesbills. CAUTION: Using this plant may bring on some side effects including nausea, vomiting and headache. Nevertheless, Native Americans used the leaves of this plant to treat stomach complaints, digestive problems and as an appetizer. The plant was also used for treating inflammation, back pain and getting rid of all kinds of worms.

Greenbriar (*Smilax bona-nox*). This plant is also known as catbrier, bullbrier, catvine or zarzaparilla. Native Americans used greenbrier as a mild diuretic and blood purifier. The Cherokee also used a tea of the roots to treat joint pain and arthritis. In addition, the bark and leaves have been combined with lard to prepare a salve that was applied to treat sores, scrapes, cuts and minor burns.

Honeysuckle (*Lonicera*). Honeysuckle is a genus of about 180 species of climbers and shrubs that come from the family *Caprifoliaceae* and that have been identified in Eurasia and North America. These species have been used by the Native Americans as a natural remedy for treating asthma. They have also been used to treat rheumatoid arthritis, mumps, hepatitis, and upper respiratory tract infections such as pneumonia.

Lavender (Lavandula angustifolia). Lavender has been used as a remedy for insomnia, depression, anxiety, headache and fatigue. The essential oil has antiseptic and anti-inflammatory properties. An infusion of this plant has been used to treat insect bites and soothe burns.

Licorice root (*Glycyrrhiza glabra*). CAUTION: avoid if pregnant or if experiencing premenstrual syndrome or if you have kidney disease or high blood pressure or if you are on any digoxin-based medication. Use with caution and only under the supervision of a licensed doctor, if you have cirrhosis of the liver. Do not use for longer than six weeks. Consuming excessive quantities may cause sluggishness, headache, potassium depletion and, in extreme cases, high blood pressure, edema or even congestive heart failure. The root of this plant is edible and may be eaten raw, but is often used as a sweetener, flavoring and in the preparation of tea. Licorice powder is extracted from the root. Glycyrrhizin, which can be found in the root, is a substance that is about fifty times sweeter than table sugar (sucrose).

Licorice protects and detoxifies the liver. It is anti-inflammatory and is used in the treatment of various conditions including mouth ulcers and arthritis. Licorice root is used in the treatment of coughs, catarrh, bronchitis, urinary tract infections and gastritis. Licorice is also ingested internally (as tea, infusion or decoction) to treat coughs, bronchitis, asthma, arthritis, allergies, peptic ulcer, stomach complaints, food poisoning, chronic fatigue and Addison's disease, etc. Externally, licorice root is used to treat eczema, herpes and shingles.

Mint (*Mentha*). Mint contains many powerful antioxidants and vitamins including vitamins A and C, potassium, magnesium, phosphorus and calcium. The Cherokee have consumed mint tea to reduce blood pressure and to stimulate the digestive system. Mint leaves were also crushed to produce ointment and salves used to treat itching and skin rashes. Mint has also been used as a bath solution and to treat stomach ache and headaches. Mint can be made into a poultice or tea. It can also be added to food or chewed raw. Mint oil is used as an energy or mood booster and it has great anti-inflammatory properties that can soothe irritated skin and treat bee stings or bug bites. Mint counteracts allergies by hindering the release of histamines which cause runny nose, hay fever and other symptoms. Mint is used in toothpastes because the menthol in mint works as an antimicrobial, killing germs that cause tooth decay and bad breath. The mint plant is easy to grow in any environment and is also used as a natural repellant against bugs.

Mullein (*Verbascum thapsus*). CAUTION: the seeds of this plant are toxic and act as a natural pesticide. This plant is also called duffle, Aaron's rod, gordolobo, lungwort, hare's beard, beggar's blanket or fluffweed. Native Americans used this plant to treat respiratory and lung challenges. The roots were burned and inhaled to clear the airways and reduce inflammation of the mucus membranes lining the respiratory tract. Mullein flowers can be prepared as tea or infusion and used as sedative or to treat migraine headaches and joint pains. Mullein been traditionally smoked lie tobacco or made into oil or poultice or tea (depending on what it was intended for) and used as medicine.

Some parts of the plant like the stems, flowers and leaves were also used for food. But note that the seeds of this plant are toxic and act as a natural pesticide. Mullein has also been used to treat breathing problems (such as bronchitis, allergies, asthma and colds). This is because the plant contains saponins which act as an expectorant. To treat cough, the Native Americans would either smoke the mullein and make it into a tea that they would drink with honey or molasses.

The presence of verbascoside in mullein makes the plant an antibacterial and an anti-inflammatory. And recent studies have confirmed mullein to be potent against all forms of staphylococcus infections. As a result, mullein is useful for treating many health complaints such as blisters, cuts, rashes, stiff joints, burns, sore muscles and arthritis. Mullein has also been used for muscle spasms, gastric disorders and menstruation cramps. The root has also been used for treating bladder infections.

Prickly pear cactus (*Opuntia focus-indica*). This plant has been used as both food as well as medicine. Native Americans prepared a poultice from the matured pads of this plant and used it as an antiseptic and for treating burns, wounds and boils. This plant has also been ingested internally as tea to boost the immune system and to treat urinary tract infections. It can also be used to reduce cholesterol and to prevent diabetes and cardiovascular disease.

Rose hip (*Rosa*). Rose hips consist of the round part of a rose flower which contains the seeds and is located below the petals. They come from the genus, *Rosa*, that comprises of about 100 species of shrubs that come from the rose family (*Rosaceae*). Rose hips are also called by the following names: Persian rose, wild rose, dog rose, wild boar fruit, hop fruit, rose hep, rose haw, hip and gulab. They contain a high amount of Vitamin C, hence they are used for preventing and treating flu, cold and related sicknesses. Rose hips have also been used to treat fever, rheumatoid arthritis, diarrhea, infections, the common cold, upset stomach and other conditions. Rose hips are also good for all kinds of stomach ailments, stomach ulcers and intestinal diseases. Native Americans have used an infusion/tea made of rose hips to rejuvenate the kidneys and the bladder. The roots of the plant have also been used to treat diarrhea. The petals of the plant have also been made into tea and used to treat sore throat.

Rosemary (*Salvia rosmarinus* formerly *Rosmarinus officinalis*). Native Americans have used rosemary as an analgesic to ease sore joint pain, muscle spasm, muscle pain and to boost the memory and enhance both the nervous and circulatory systems. Rosemary also works for indigestion.

Sage (*Salvia officinalis*). CAUTION: sage has been found to be toxic when taken for the long-term or when taken in excess. Nevertheless, sage has been used by Native Americans to purify, cleanse and detoxify the body. They have also used it to treat colds, the flu, cuts, bruises, spasms and abdominal cramps, etc. The Navajo have used sage to treat diabetes. Sage has also been used effectively as a natural remedy for toothaches (although it is considered as temporary remedy). The dried leaves or fresh leaves of this plant have been prepared as tea and poured in the mouth to ease tooth aches and pains. Sage poultice has also been placed on or close to an inflamed and painful area around the mouth (teeth, mouth or cheek) to relieve the pain. Native Americans have also used sage as aromatherapy by burning it around the house to mask unpleasant odors.

Saw Palmetto (*Serenoa repens*). CAUTION: Avoid this plant if you are using hormonal drugs. Avoid during pregnancy and lactation. Take with food. Rare adverse effects include: gastrointestinal symptoms and mild headache. It may diminish libido in males and may increase blood pressure and the possibility of back pain. The native tribes of Florida, such as the Seminoles, were known to have consumed this plant for food while their healers also used it as a natural cure for stomach complaints. The plant was also used as an appetizer, to reduce inflammation and to aid digestion.

Saw palmetto berries are used to treat urinary tract problems and prostate problems. The berries also make a good tonic. The ripe (but partially dried fruit) has been used as an aphrodisiac, an expectorant, an antiseptic, a tonic, a diuretic and a sedative. Saw palmetto is taken internally to treat debility in elderly men, to treat impotence, absent or reduced sex drive, testicular atrophy, prostate enlargement, bronchial issues and wasting diseases. It is also used to stimulate breast enlargement in women.

Saw palmetto also strengthens and builds body tissue and stimulates weight gain. A tincture or the fruit pulp is given to those suffering from general debility or wasting disease. The fruit also helps to strengthen the neck of the bladder, treat coughs, colds, asthma and irritated mucous membranes, etc. A suppository made of powdered saw palmetto fruits in cocoa butter, has been used as a vaginal and uterine tonic. This plant can be found around

South-eastern North America, from South Carolina to Florida, west to Arkansas).

Slippery Elm (*Ulmus rubra*). CAUTION: Outer bark has caused abortions. Avoid, if pregnant. This tree can be found in central and southern North America (from Maine to Florida to Texas to North Dakota). The leaves, fruit and inner bark of this tree are edible. The leaves and the inner bark can be eaten cooked or raw. They can be dried, ground and powdered and used as a soup thickener or mixed with flour to make bread. The inner bark can also be used to prepare a tea. And the young fruit can be eaten cooked or raw.

Slippery elm bark is useful for treating chest mucous membrane irritations, stomach, intestinal and urinary issues and the tree is also included in the popular Essiac formula used for cancer treatment. The inner bark is used to treat sore throats, stomach ulcers, indigestion and digestive irritation. It has also been externally applied to burns, scalds and fresh wounds. The whole bark has been utilized as a mechanical irritant to cause abortions and so has now been banned in many countries.

Sumac (*Rhus*). Sumac is a genus of approximately 35 species of plants, shrubs and small trees that come from the cashew family. Sumac is a spice and has many health benefits. Native Americans made a decoction from its bark to cure sore throat and diarrhea. An infusion or tea of its leaves were also used for treating fever. The fresh leaves were mixed with berries to form a paste that was used against poison ivy.

Uva ursi (*Arctostaphylos uva-ursi*). This plant is also called beargrape or bearberry, perhaps, because the fruit of this plant is especially loved by bears. CAUTION: this plant contains arbutin which may be toxic if ingested in high quantities. Ingestion of large quantities of this plant may trigger allergic reactions, nausea and even seizures. Also, avoid this plant if you are pregnant or breastfeeding or if you have kidney or liver disease. Nevertheless, the Blackfeet Nation have used this plant primarily as food, to make jelly and as seasoning. Generally, Native Americans used uva ursi to treat bladder disorders and urinary tract infections. Teas made from the plant and extracts of the leaves have also been used as laxatives and diuretics. This plant is considered by some to be an astringent and to be able to cure sexually transmitted diseases, but good evidence from clinical studies do not exist to substantiate these claims.

Valerian (*Valeriana officinalis*). CAUTION: Valerian should not be used for more than 3 weeks at a time without being followed by a break of the same duration, as continual use of more than 3 weeks without a break may cause headache and depression. Also for about 7% of the population, Valerian may cause an opposite effect (that is, cause restlessness, giddiness, agitation and sleeplessness). Also do not use valerian with children. Nevertheless, the root of this plant is medicinally very potent and is used to treat anxiety and insomnia. An infusion/tea is made of the plant and consumed to treat muscle spasm, cramps, bowel irritations and gastrointestinal disorders. The simplest way to prepare valerian is to decoct the root and ingest the decoction as needed.

Wild black cherry (*Prunus serotina*). This plant is also known as wild cherry or chokecherry. CAUTION: The leaves and seeds of this plant are poisonous! Handle with care. The bark and the fruit of this plant are edible and are used medicinally. The bark is made into a tea and used to treat the flu, colds, coughs, bronchitis, laryngitis, sore throat, asthma, swollen lymph nodes, high blood pressure, and arthritis, among other ailments. It is also used as a mild sedative and an appetite stimulant. The Mohegans allowed the fruit to ferment naturally for about a year before using it to treat dysentery.

Wild ginger (colic root/heart- leaf-leaf). This plant is also known as big stretch, colic root, cat's foot or heart-leaf). CAUTION: The US Food and Drug Administration (FDA) has warned that this plant is nephrotoxic and that it contains aristolochic acid (a carcinogen). Furthermore, note that this plant is called "wild ginger" simply because its rhizomes smell and taste like the more widely-known "ginger root". But the two plants are not the same and they are not particularly related. Nevertheless, Native Americans have used wild ginger to treat several ailments. The Cherokee, for instance, drank an infusion of this plant to help digestion. Wild Ginger is also known to be effective against gas, bloating, stomach cramps, colic and aches. The plant is also useful for removal of excess mucus from the lungs. The plant is also effective for the treatment of ear infection and ear ache. The roots of the plant can also be used to prevent nausea and combat bronchial infections.

Wild rose (*Rosa acicularis*). The hips of this flower are quite high in vitamin A and vitamin C. Native Americans used this plant to prevent and to treat the common cold. This rose species is the most abundant of all the rose species of the boreal forest in northern North America. It is native to the northern Great Plains in the United States (that is, east of the Rocky Mountains and west of the Mississippi River). And it is the official flower of the province of Alberta, Canada. This flower blooms beginning May and continuing up to July, annually. An infusion/tea of this plant was used as a mild diuretic and taken to stimulate the bladder and the kidneys. An infusion of the petals of this flower was also taken to treat sore throat.

Willow (*Salix*). Willow is a genus of trees and shrubs that come from the family *Salicaceae*. But one compound that is common to all the species under this willow genus (*Salix*) is salicin, the source of acetylsalicylic acid or aspirin. Both salicin and aspirin combat fever and relieve pains as a result of their anti-inflammatory ingredients. The bark is the more medicinally potent part of this tree. Members of this genus have a high quantity of flavonoids that are anti-inflammatory in nature. Within this genus, the specie of willow with the highest salicin includes purple willow, crack willow and white willow. To enjoy the medicinal benefits of willow, boil the bark and consume as tea.

Witch hazel (*Hamamelis viginiana*). This plant has astringent and anti-inflammation properties. It is found in many parts of the United States and also in southern Canada. This plant is generally used for the treatment of bruises, swellings, bug bites and muscle pain. It has also been used to stop bleeding and to treat sunburn, hemorrhoids, eczema, varicose veins, acne and poison ivy skin problems.

Yarrow (*Achillea millefolium*). This plant is also known as nosebleed plant, thousand-leaf, squirrel tail, Saloli gatoga, devil's nettle, old man's repper and thousand-seal). Yarrow has been used to treat blood clotting disorder because it can help wounds form scabs and easily heal. If taken with water, it can function to eliminate intestinal and digestive-related inflammation. Cherokee medicine men used this plant for different ailments. The crushed fresh leaves of this plant can be used as a poultice to stop fresh-wound from bleeding. An infusion or tea of this plant is effective for stopping or slowing internal bleeding. In addition, the tea can aid digestion and enhance the function of gallbladder and kidneys. A decoction of the stems and leaves can also be used as a form of astringent for treating acne and other skin infections.

CHAPTER 6: NATIVE AMERICAN HERBAL CURES AND REMEDIES FOR DENTAL HEALTH

Antimicrobials for oral health

Echinacea, Coneflower (*Echinacea purpurea*). Echinacea has been used by Native Americans as an antibacterial, antiviral, and antifungal. Echinacea has also been used as an immune-system stimulant. It also helps to fight the common cold and flu. Echinacea helps the immune system to fight off whatever germs that could cause sore throat or dental/oral infections and decay. Echinacea is best used for dental health as a gargle.

Myrrh (*Commiphora myrrha*). CAUTION: People with kidney diseases should avoid using myrrh. Also myrrh can become toxic in the body after prolonged or excessive use. Nevertheless, this herb has potent antiseptic ingredients and it has been used in Native American herbology to treat various mouth infections. You can add myrrh to a few drops of water and then apply the solution to mouth sores with a cotton swab, for relief. Because of the astringent in myrrh, it is able to reduce inflammation and fight off bacterial infection. So it is good to rinse the mouth with an infusion of myrrh leaves frequently, as part of good oral hygiene. To do so, simmer a teaspoon of powdered myrrh in a cup or two of water, stir thoroughly and rinse your mouth with the solution, about five times daily.

Honey. Pure honey is one of the everyday natural remedies used by Native Americans for health purposes and which is still used today. The innate peroxide in honey ranks it among the best antiviral and antibacterial natural products available. Honey helps to heal wounds (both outside and inside the mouth). Honey acts as a barrier, preventing infection and moisturizing wounds while they heal. Today, the use of honey as a salve helps to heal canker sores and minor tongue and gum sores.

Toothaches

Western Yarrow or Common Yarrow (*Achillea millefolium*). Several Native American tribes (such as the Carrier, the Cree, Woodlands, the Okanagan-Colville, the Paiute, the Costanoan and the Saanich tribes, etc.) used this plant as a toothache remedy. They either crushed the root of the plant and placed it on the tooth or took a decoction of the root or chewed the plant's leaves for toothache relief.

Thyme (Thymus vulgaris). This plant is also called garden thyme, common thyme, German thyme, French thyme, English thyme, winter thyme or summer thyme. CAUTION: Avoid overuse of thyme essential oil. Because it is concentrated (as an essential oil) and so can be unsafe in excess doses. Also do not use if pregnant or breastfeeding. Nevertheless, Native Americans have used this herb to relieve all sorts of pain, sprains and aches. Thyme oil, the essential oil of thyme (Thymus vulgaris), contains between 20% to 54% thymol as well as other essential compounds. Thymol is an antiseptic and is used as an active ingredient in many commercially-produced mouthwashes (e.g. Listerine). Thyme oil has also been used to aid enhanced flow of blood to the surface of the skin. The oil can also be applied to toothaches for relief. Thyme is also used externally to treat tonsillitis and gum disease. Thyme is strongly antioxidant and its regular use enhances the longevity and health of the individual cells of the body (including the cells of the tooth, mouth and tongue). The whole thyme plant is also used to treat many ailments including sore throats.

Redshank, Ribbonwod (*Adenostoma sparsifolium*).
This plant was used by the Diegueno Indians as a toothache remedy. They used an infusion of the plant as a mouthwash to aid toothache relief.

Calamus (*Acorus calamus*). The Blackfoot Indians used this plant as a toothache remedy. They applied a poultice of the crushed roots of this plant, plus some hot water to an aching tooth for toothache relief. The Chippewa Indians used the plant as a pediatric dental aid. They gave children a decoction of the root of this plant or the dried root of the plant to be chewed by children for relief from toothache. And the Iroquois Indians packed the root of the plant into the cavity in a tooth to break up the ailing tooth or smoked the root of the plant and sucked the smoke into the cavity in the tooth for toothache relief.

Garlic (*Allium sativum*). Garlic has strong antibacterial, antiviral and antifungal properties. It is a natural anesthetic and will give pain relief to the area of the body to which it is applied. Garlic is also a natural broad-spectrum antibiotic. And here's one important thing to note: while bacteria may eventually build resistance against many modern pharmaceutical antibiotics, bacteria are unable to build resistance against garlic (regardless of how regularly or how much you use garlic). This quality therefore makes garlic a very effective natural antibiotic. The poultice or paste of garlic has been used to relieve toothaches. And the repeated application of crushed raw garlic to an abscessed tooth can drastically reduce or eliminate the infection in that abscessed tooth. (But despite your use of any alternative treatment, be sure to consult your dentist regarding an abscessed tooth).

To get quick toothache relief, crush a clove of garlic, add a little pinch of salt to the mash, then apply the mashed garlic to any painful part of the tooth. Leave on for several minutes, then rinse out with warm salt water. Alternatively, you can chew some cloves of garlic twice daily. Chew the cloves with the affected tooth to maximize contact with the garlic juice. Finally rinse out your mouth with warm salt water. And if there is too much swelling and inflammation, especially around the jaw area and you need to fight the tooth infection from inside, you can do the following: crush or finely chop 3 or 4 cloves of raw garlic, mix the garlic into a cup of plain yoghurt and enjoy! Taking garlic internally will help you to fight the infection from inside and reduce the inflammation more quickly.

Sage (*Salvia officinalis*). Sage is another evergreen herb that is quite effective for treating teeth and gum complaints and maintaining oral health. Sage has been noted to possess strong astringent, antiseptic, spasmolytic and aromatic properties and noted to be effective for the treatment of gum infection/inflammation, dental abscesses, mouth ulcers and throat infections, etc. Sage contains over 60 beneficial essential compounds and other properties, that combat various types of health problems, including dental and oral health issues. Sage is especially good for gum disease and because of its anti-inflammatory properties, it helps to significantly decrease gum inflammation.

Sage also has powerful antimicrobial, antibacterial, antiviral and antifungal properties that neutralize dental-plaque-causing microbes and cavity-causing bacteria. Sage also has compounds that accelerate wound healing thus making it a wonderful remedy for swollen, sore and bleeding gums. Several studies have confirmed the effectiveness of sage against cavity-causing bacteria and for healing gum and teeth complaints. One such study has shown that a sage-based mouthwash kills one of the principal bacteria that causes dental plaque and cavities (*Streptococcus mutans*). The essential oil of sage has also been shown to kill the cavity-linked fungus *Candida albicans*.

The best way to use sage for dental applications is to prepare it as a tea. You may use dried or fresh sage to make the tea. Boil water. Add sage leaves to the boiling water. Turn off heat and allow the leaves to simmer until the water is cool enough to drink.

Strain off the leaves and pour the remaining liquid into a cup. Your sage tea is ready! Swish the tea around inside your mouth for 30 seconds to 1 minute at a time, and spit. A tea made from 2 tablespoons of fresh or dried sage leaves will provide relief from toothache and swollen or sore gums.

Alternatively, you may place a warm, wet sage tea bag on the affected gum or teeth for relief. Also, alternatively you may prepare your own sage mouth rinse using sage essential oil. It is just as effective. Indeed, sage essential oil has been shown to have strong antimicrobial, antibacterial, antiviral and antifungal properties. And sage essential oil is equally effective against disease-causing oral/dental microbes. It is also strongly preventive against gum diseases. To create your own sage oil mouth rinse, add 3 drops of sage essential oil to 1 cup of water. Brush your teeth thoroughly, then pour some of the rinse inside your mouth and swish vigorously around inside your mouth, then spit.

A poultice made of sage leaves may also be placed on or close to the affected area in the mouth, for relief.

Clove (*Syzygium aromaticum*). CAUTION: the use of cloves may trigger adverse effects if ingested orally by people with immune system and blood clotting disorders, liver problems or food allergies. Nevertheless, the mostly-used medicinal part of the clove tree is the flower bud. Native Americans have used clove oil (the essential oil of clove) which contains eugenol as an analgesic for dental pain relief (among other uses). Eugenol constitutes between 72% and 90% of the essential oil of clove. Clove oil (eugenol as the active ingredient) has been used against many types of pain including toothache pain. Eugenol has also been combined with zinc oxide to treat alveolar osteitis. Clove oil and cloves are used safely today as active ingredients in toothpastes. Even in modern dentistry, clove oil is generally used as a local antiseptic and as an analgesic. And eugenol is widely used in modern dentistry for its antianaerobic bacterial and anesthetic properties. Clove stings upon application but brings pain relief afterwards. Clove oil, though volatile, can be applied directly on the spot of the toothache.

Ginger (*Zingiber officinale*). In Native American medicine, ginger root was roasted and used to cover a sore tooth to bring relief to toothache. Sometimes the ginger root was chewed with the affected tooth/teeth (where possible), thus generating saliva which carries the active ingredients from the ginger root into the affected tooth, bringing relief.

Ginger is highly effective for maintaining oral health and hygiene. Ginger contains anti-inflammatory, anti-bacterial, anti-viral and anti-oxidant properties. Together these properties form a powerful defense against all sorts of dental diseases. Ginger has been found to be effective for various oral concerns including: toothaches, bad breath, halitosis, cavities, plaques, gum protection and gingivitis or even periodontitis. The gingerol in ginger works to counteract bad breath and kills the germs that cause cavities. Ginger also has an active ingredient (Raffinose) which prevents the accumulation of bacteria on enamel, which is what leads to the formation and build-up of plaque. Indeed, the consumption of ginger protects both the teeth and the gums as well.

Here are some of the ways you may use ginger for your oral health. You may eat ginger raw, as cooked ginger may have lost some of its properties. Wash your fresh and raw ginger root thoroughly under running water. Dry it a, then scrape off or cut off the outer skin of ginger root. Cut the root into smaller pieces and chew some pieces with the affected tooth. The toothache will significantly reduce. You can also add ginger to your meals (for example as part of your salad). Or in pastries, bread, as spice for cooking, etc. And you may also ingest ginger as tea. Indeed, drinking ginger as tea is the commonest way through which many people consume ginger for health. Ginger as tea is also particularly good for relieving sore throat. To make a cup of ginger tea, peel and cut some fresh ginger roots into small pieces. Put into boiling water for some minutes. Strain into a mug. Wait until the tea is cool. And your ginger tea is ready!

Chamomile (*Marticaria recutita* or *Chamaemelum nobile*). Chamomile contains several terpenoids and flavonoids which have been shown to be anti-inflammatory, antimicrobial and antispasmodic. Native Americans often put a warm poultice of chamomile on a sore tooth or on the outside of the cheek near the sore tooth, to obtain relief. Chamomile is also effective against receding gums. In one scientific study, study participants (who had bleeding gums and gingivitis) rinsed their mouths with chamomile extract, twice a day, for 15 days. At the end of the 15 days it was found that the gum bleeding had been reduced by the chamomile extract. In addition, it was discovered that the chamomile also had antimicrobial effects as it significantly diminished pathogenic oral bacteria activity. By the way, the reduced bacteria populations included *Streptococcus sangus* and *Streptococcus mitis*. These two bacteria are known to cause pain, inflammation and bleeding in the gums, teeth and mouth.

One way to use chamomile for oral health is to create your own chamomile mouth rinse. To do so, add some powdered chamomile into a cup of hot water. You may also add a little lemon juice and/or vanilla extract (its' up to you). Then brush your teeth and after brushing, pour some of the chamomile mouth rinse into your mouth and swish it around inside your mouth. Spit it out when finished. Due to the antibacterial and anti-inflammatory properties in chamomile, this rinse will soothe dental swelling and combat oral germs.

Anise (*Pimpinella anisum*). CAUTION: pregnant women should not medicinally use Anise seeds, although regular culinary amounts are safe. Anise seeds have been chewed to help alleviate toothaches. Drinking Anise-seed tea (prepared from anise seeds) improves digestion, coughs, and eased headaches. Anise-seed tea is made by crushing some anise seeds, steeping them for 10 minutes in boiling water and straining out the seeds. Anise oil is also an antiseptic and is beneficial to dental/oral health.

Anise oil helps in the re-mineralization that is necessary for a healthy mouth. Anise seeds have long been used as a natural breath freshener. Anise tea (which is made from Anise seeds) also naturally freshens the breath. Anise tea also generally promotes and protects oral health. This is because it contains some natural antiseptic properties that help to keep bacteria levels in check, acts as a natural mouth rinse and gets rid of bacterial infections.

Marjoram (Origanum majorana). A somewhat related specie to marjoram is "oregano" (Origanum vulgare) also referred to as "wild marjoram" and sometimes mistakenly listed as Origanum majorana. Marjoram has been used to soothe toothaches. Drops of the essential oil of marjoram have been placed directly into cavities of teeth to obtain relief. The essential oil of marjoram is antimicrobial and antibacterial and has been found to act against Staphylococcus aureus, so makes a good mouthwash or mouth rinse.

Swelling and bleeding

Spotted Geranium (*Geranium maculatum*). This plant is also called the wild geranium, wood geranium, wild cranesbill or spotted cranesbill, alum bloom, alum root or old maid's nightcap. Spotted Geranium is a perennial plant native to eastern North America (from southwestern Quebec to southern Manitoba to Georgia and Alabama to South Dakota and Oklahoma). Spotted geranium has been used in herbal medicine, and is considered an astringent, a substance that stops bleeding and causes tissues to contract. The Meskwaki Indians used this plant for oral care. An infusion of root of the plant was used to treat toothache, sore gums and aching teeth.

Blueberries (*Vaccinium myrtillus*). CAUTION: A serving of blueberries contains approximately 10 grams of sugar. Therefore, eating excess quantities of blueberries or eating blueberries too often, can put your teeth at risk because of the sugar. So, the key is moderation. Nevertheless, blueberries have been described as a natural weapon against tooth decay. Eating a handful of blueberries per day have been reported to be able to help reduce oral health issues. Indeed, studies have found that blueberries can reduce the risk of tooth decay by lowering the activity of bacteria in the mouth. Blueberries are a good source of polyphenols, antioxidants that protect the body against free radicals and fight bacteria (including the bacteria that causes plaque). Blueberries can be eaten raw, by themselves or together with other foods such as yoghurt or cereal. Blueberries can be used to make a mouthwash or a paste. This can be applied to an inflamed gum for pain/inflammation relief. You can use the blueberry mouthwash to rinse your mouth about three times per day.

Stevia (*Stevia rebaudiana*). The leaves of this plant are known to be very sweet. In fact, stevia (in whole leaf form) is about 30 times sweeter than table sugar (sucrose) but once the stevia has been refined, it is almost 300 times sweeter that table sugar. So, stevia is used as a sugar substitute or sweetener. Stevia is used in low-carb diets because it has zero calories and has very tiny, almost insignificant, effect on blood glucose levels. With regard to oral health, glycosides, a compound in stevia has been found to be effective against tooth decay, cavities and plaque. Studies (in vitro) have shown that stevia extracts have antibacterial properties that are active against the multiplication of mouth bacteria including those bacteria that are associated with plaques (e.g. *Streptococcus sobrinus*, *Streptococcus mutans*, and *Lactobacillus acidophilus*). Thus that stevia helps prevent tooth decay. Many of today's toothpastes contain stevia as an active ingredient. To use stevia, add a few fresh stevia leaves to tea. Dried stevia leaves can also be powdered and used to make other edibles such as sauces, desserts and soups.

Witch Hazel (*amamelis virginiana*). Native to North America, witch hazel can be found in southern Canada and the eastern and Midwestern United States. Witch hazel has been one of the Native Americans' folk remedies for dental health. A cloth soaked in witch-hazel tea is placed on the troubled spot. The with-hazel tea is considered effective for reducing swelling and controlling bleeding after tooth extractions.

Arnica (*Arnica montana*). Other names for this herb include common arnica, leopard's bane, mountain daisy, mountain tobacco and wolfsbane, etc. CAUTION: Arnica should never be used internally or used on open sores or wounds. Also, arnica should not be used for a prolonged time. Prolonged or excessive use may cause edema, allergies, bladder condition or inflammatory skin reactions. Pregnant and breastfeeding women should use arnica only under the supervision of a licensed doctor or other healthcare provider.

Nevertheless, Arnica has been used traditionally to speed the healing of tissues and as a remedy for various ailments. The herb has also been proven to hasten the healing of sores or wounds around mouth. The herb is rarely administered in a pure form or used as an herbal tea, rather it is mostly administered in ointments, oils, tinctures, gels and homeopathic forms. Arnica is used for sore mouth, sore throat and pain after the extraction of wisdom tooth, etc. Arnica is also applied to the skin for pain, swelling, aches, bruises, sprains, arthritis, rheumatism, leg ulcers (in diabetic patients), insect bites, acne and chapped lips, etc. Arnica is antibacterial and effective against listeria and salmonella. It is also an anti-inflammatory and helps to absorb internal bleeding back into the body.

To make oil the essential oil of arnica, for every 5 parts of extra virgin olive oil, use 1 part of arnica flowers. To make an arnica extract, add 2 grams of fresh or dried arnica flowers to 1 deciliter of boiling water. Strain for approximately 10 minutes. Use extract as a gargle or as a wrap. To make an arnica tincture, add 30 grams of dried arnica flower preserved in 30 milliliters of food-grade alcohol.

Calendula (*Calendula officinalis*). This plant is also called by the following names: the pot marigold, Scotch marigold, common marigold or ruddles. Calendula officianalis has been shown to have anti-inflammatory, anti-viral, antibacterial, antifungal and anti-genotoxic properties, in vitro. It has also been found to possess astringent properties (despite not having a high tannin content). The tea or juice of this plant can be used as mouthwash for soothing, healing and soothing sensitive gums. Swishing plus diluted tea has been confirmed to relieve sensitive and tender gums. The leaves can also be made into a poultice that can help prevent infection and help cuts and scratches to heal faster.

Mint (*Mentha*). Mint contains many powerful antioxidants and vitamins including vitamins A, C, potassium, magnesium, phosphorus and calcium. Mint can be made into a poultice, ointment, salve or tea. It can also be added to food or chewed raw. Mint is used in toothpastes because its menthol constituent works as an antimicrobial, killing germs that cause tooth decay and bad breath. Mint tea mixed with egg yolk has also been used as a gargle to relieve sensitive gums.

Bloodroot (*Sanguinaria Canadensis*). Bloodroot can be found in North America from Canada (Nova Scotia) to Florida to the Mississippi embayment and the Great Lakes. CAUTION: Bloodroot root is toxic. Consuming it in excessive quantities causes nausea, vomiting and a depression of the central nervous system. In extreme cases, it may be fatal. Avoid using this plant if pregnant or breastfeeding. Nevertheless, bloodroot has been used to prepare toothpastes and mouthwashes. Sanguinarine is the name of the primary active compound in bloodroot and it is effective in preventing plaque formation. Indeed, sanguinarine is used as a dental-plaque inhibitor. Sanguinarine has been approved by the

United States Food and Drugs Administration (FDA) for inclusion in toothpastes as an anti-plaque or antibacterial ingredient. However, note that sanguinaria in oral care products is associated with premalignant oral leukoplakia.

Externally, the sap of the fresh bloodroot root or an infusion of the root has been used to treat several ailments including sore throats. An infusion of the root or root is used. To make a bloodroot mouthwash, add 1 teaspoon of pulverized bloodroot some spearmint leaves in water. Stir thoroughly, then strain properly. The remaining solution is your bloodroot mouthwash and it's very effective for oral care.

Vervain (*Verbena officinalis*). This flowering plant is also known by the following names: common verbena, wild verbena, blue vervain, wild hyssop, Indian hyssop, enchanter's plant, simpler's joy, juno's tears, mosquito plant, pigeon weed, pigeon's grass, holy herb or herb of the cross. Vervain has become naturalized in North America. CAUTION. Vervain is not suitable in pregnancy because it stimulates the uterus and triggers labor-inducing effects. So, vervain should be avoided by pregnant and breastfeeding women. Also avoid ingesting this herb in large quantities. Nevertheless, Native American tribes have used the root of this plant to treat throat inflammation and swelling, gum and tooth infections/inflammation and ulcers; It has also been used to treat circulatory issues, headaches and insomnia.

Vervain is anti-inflammatory, antibacterial and astringent, etc. Vervain's natural astringent properties are makes it an effective oral rinse for mouth ulcers and bleeding gums. Vervain mouth rinse will also relieve inflammation and sore throat. Vervain can be used as an infusion/tea, ointment, tincture or topically. However, vervain's traditional medicinal application is as tea (although the vervain flavor is particularly bitter). Vervain can also be made into a skin lotion or a compress.

Aphthous ulcers

Goldenseal (*Hydrastis canadensis*). Native Americans used this herb as tea or ground it to powder to make a poultice. The tea made from this plant and the powder (poultice) can be applied to the surface of the affected tooth or gum. Goldenseal can be used to treat canker sores and gum.

Licorice (*Glycyrrhiza glabra* and *Glycyrrhiza uralensis*). CAUTION: avoid licorice if you have high blood pressure. Nevertheless, Glycyrrhizol A, the active compound in licorice has strong anti-inflammatory antimicrobial, antibacterial, antifungal and antiviral properties and so helps to prevent the buildup of mouth bacteria, acts against gum disease and cavities and soothes mouth ulcers. Licorice is also active against all discomfort associated with aphthous ulcers. To use licorice for oral health, massage licorice powder into your gums and teeth or chew on a licorice root (if possible with the affected tooth or in the affected side of your mouth).

Figs (*Ficus carica*). Fig is also called edible fig, cultivated fig, common fig and wild fig. This specie is native to western Asia and the Middle East and has become naturalized across North America. CAUTION: Eating fig fruits might trigger allergy symptoms in sensitive people. The symptoms may include itching of the mucus membranes and the skin, vomiting and diarrhea. So, do not eat figs if you have a fig allergy. Also, avoid consuming figs a minimum of 2 weeks before a scheduled surgery. To treat a gum boil, dip a thin strip of dried fig fruit in milk before you toast it, then place it on the swollen gum while hot. The roasted fig fruit is emollient and has also been used as a poultice to treat dental abscesses. To treat a sore throat, drink a hot infusion made of boiled crushed fig leaves and olive pit. Or gargle with a decoction of fig fruits to relieve sore throat. Fig leaves and fig fruit may be pulverized together and used to make a gargle that can relieve sore throat. And to treat toothache, hold a fig in your mouth or place a fig against the affected tooth or swish fig juice around the affected tooth. If there is a cavity in the tooth, ensure that the fig juice enters into the cavity.

Sore throats

Western White Clematis (*Clematis ligusticifolia*). This plant is also called yerba de chiva (goatbeard plant), pipestems, peppervine, old-man's beard, deciduous traveler's-joy, creekside virgin's bower, western white virgin's bower or creek clematis. This plant can be found in western North America, in Washington and southern British Columbia, also in northwest Mexico and California.

The leaves and stems of this plant (which are peppery to the taste) have been chewed for sore throats and colds. The Montana Indians have particularly chewed this plant to treat sore throat. A poultice or an infusion of this plant has also been applied to wounds, sores, swellings, and bruises and also used to treat backaches and chest pain.

Salt (*sodium chloride*). Salt is also known as table salt or common salt. Salt (as salt water gargle) is a great ingredient for soothing sore throats and clearing the throat of any mucus or congestion. But salt water does not actually cure a sore throat. It only helps to ease the pain of a sore throat. Most sore throats are viral and not bacterial and will go away by themselves in 3 days to 1 week. Gargling with salt water as you wait for the sore throat to go away is just a way to help alleviate the pain of the sore throat, as you wait. A good salt water gargle for sore throat must be hypertonic. That means that it has to have enough salt in it to make the solution have a higher osmotic pressure than the fluid in the cells in your mouth (so that the salt water will be able to draw the fluid in the cells in your mouth, along with the viruses and bacteria in your mouth, to the surface). In other words, your salt water gargle for sore throat has to be very salty to work.

To make a good salt water gargle for sore throat, add a ¼
teaspoon of salt into a 1/2 cup of warm water and stir thoroughly. The water should be warm so as to increase the flow of blood to your throat and activate your immune system. You may gargle up to 2 to 4 times per day until the sore throat is gone.

But be sure to be drinking much water during the same period to prevent the salt water from drying out your mouth. CAUTION: avoid the salt water gargle if you have high blood pressure.

Ginger (*Zingiber officinale*). Ginger is highly effective for maintaining oral health and hygiene. Ginger contains anti-inflammatory, anti-bacterial, anti-viral and anti-oxidant properties. Together these properties form a powerful defense against all sorts of dental diseases. Ginger is good at relieving inflamed tonsils and sore throats especially if you gargle with the juice or tea. To make a cup of ginger tea, peel and cut some fresh ginger roots into small pieces. Put into boiling water for some minutes. Strain into a mug. Wait until the tea is cool. And your ginger tea is ready. You may drink it as tea or use it as a gargle with which to wash your mouth. Both uses are effective against sore throat.

Beets (*Beta vulgaris*). This plant has been confirmed to be effective against sore throat. Beetroot has been combined with vinegar and honey or sage and used as a remedy for colds and sore throat. Beetroot juice is also considered an aphrodisiac. The mineral, boron, in beetroot actually plays a vital role in the production of the sex hormones.

Cayenne pepper is a variety of *Capsicum annuum*. This plant is very effective against sore throat if used as a gargle (the crushed fruit mixed with water). A cayenne pepper gargle is able to provide sore throat pain relief for up to 2 hours. It is thought that certain compounds contained in cayenne pepper are able to obstruct the peptide that communicates pain signals to the brain, therefore providing pain relief. To make a cayenne pepper gargle, mix 2 teaspoons of powdered cayenne pepper into ½ cup of hot water. Stir thoroughly and gargle with the solution. You may add I tablespoon of salt to the mixture as salt will also help to ease the sore throat pain.

Sauerkraut juice. Sauerkraut juice is the naturally fermented juice of the cabbage plant. Sauerkraut juice (the traditional, homemade, naturally fermented sauerkraut, not commercial sauerkraut) is effective against *sore throat*. It is also effective against *canker sores*. And there have been anecdotal reports that it quickens up the healing time for *cold sores*.

To treat sore throat, slowly sip a glass of sauerkraut juice 2 or 3 times in the day. Or gargle with sauerkraut juice morning and night and swallow it. Either of these methods can provide rapid relief to your sore throat.

To treat canker sores, take a tablespoon of sauerkraut juice in your mouth and swish it around twice a day (morning and night), then swallow it. This can also provide rapid relief and cause the canker sore to quickly go away.

To treat cold sores, at the first sign of the beginning of a cold sore, rub some sauerkraut juice on the tingling spot, and do this several times a day. In under 1 week, the cold sore should be gone. The sauerkraut juice speeds up the healing process!

To make homemade, naturally-fermented sauerkraut, do the following: chop cabbage leaves and knead some salt into them. Cover the salted cabbage leaves with a piece of clean cloth and weigh it down tightly with heavy plates or a stone. Allow to ferment for at least 6 weeks, then draw off the sauerkraut juice as needed.

Periodontal disease, caries and inflammation

California Buckeye (*Aesculus californica*) this plant was used by the Costanoan Indians and the Mendocino Indians as a toothache remedy. The Costanoans used a decoction of the bark for loose teeth and toothaches, while the Mendocino placed the bark in the cavity of an ailing tooth for relief.

Common Yarrow (Achillea millefolium). The Mahuna Indians used this plant as a toothache remedy. They inserted rolled leaves of this plant into the cavity in a painful tooth for relief.

Wild Sarsaparilla (Aralia nudicaulis). The Cree, Woodlands Indians used this plant as a pediatric oral aid. A decoction of the plant's roots is used to wash the infected gums of a teething child in order to prevent the spread of infection.

Virginia Strawberry (Fragaria virginiana). The Cherokee Indians used this fruit for dental care. They would place and hold the fruit in the mouth in order to remover tartar from the teeth.

Idaho Hymenopappus (Hymenopappus filifolius). The Hopi Indians used this plant for dental care. The root of the plant was chewed to treat decaying teeth.

Shrubby Blackberry (*Rubus fruticosus*). The roots of shrubby blackberry have been used to alleviate the loose teeth that often results from periodontal disease. The chopped roots of the shrubby blackberry are boiled in vinegar for about half an hour. Then the liquid is used to gargle and wash the loose teeth, three times a day. Supposedly, after three weeks, the loose teeth would no longer be shaky.

Oneseed Juniper (*Juniperus monosperma*). This plant was used by the Tewa Indians as a dental remedy. The gum from the plant was used as a filling for cavities and decayed teeth.

Northern Red Oak (Quercus rubra). The Mahuna Indians and the Costanoan Indians used this plant as a dental health remedy. They used juice from the plant to straighten and set loose teeth.

Lavender (Lavandula angustifolia). Gargling with lavender water has also been used to preserve loose teeth. Drop some lavender buds/ flowers in a pot of boiling water. Let the bud/flowers steep until the water cools. Then strain the buds/flowers from the cool water. The now-cooled water may be used by one suffering from loose teeth to gargle. This is claimed to preserve loose teeth.

Broadleaf Ironweed (*Vernonia glauca*). The Cherokee Indians used this plant as a dental health remedy. They used an infusion of the root of this plant for loose teeth.

CHAPTER 7: NATIVE AMERICAN HERBAL SECRETS FOR BEAUTY AND PERSONAL CARE

Native Americans have long been known as experts who possess many herbal secrets for beauty and personal care. Because Native Americans lived sustainably, off the land, they were compelled to develop an expertise in using whatever nature provided to them, to meet their beauty, personal care and healing needs. Here are some of the herbal secrets that came out of that expertise and which you may now use to help you look your best, naturally.

Personal hygiene: the secrets of cold water

The benefits of cold water

Bathing in cold water is stimulating and makes you to shiver and sweat. It also makes you tough.

Skin issues

For faster wound healing, hydrating the skin, soothing itches and irritation and soothing sunburn

Use Aloe Vera gel to fasten wound healing, hydrate your skin, soothe skin irritation, itches and sunburn. Aloe helps the skin to retain moisture. It also contains plenty anti-oxidants and phytosterols and it is antibacterial, antimicrobial, anti-inflammatory and antifungal.

For moisturizing and softening the skin and for healing skin conditions

Use agave (the tequila plant, a desert plant). Agave nectar is antibacterial and antimicrobial and when mixed with salt will heal skin conditions. The sugars in agave also moisturize and soften the skin.

For repairing and restoring mature or damaged skin

Eat prickly pear and use the oil from its seeds to help strengthen skin. Prickly pear oil is rich in vitamin E and contains many fatty acids and proteins. It nourishes and hydrates depleted, dry skin and it minimizes wrinkles, including hyper-pigmentation. It also firms the skin resulting in a lifted, look. This makes it a great remedy for mature and damaged skin. Its constituent oleic and linoleic fatty acids also help moisturize, soften and reinstate skin elasticity. Also, prickly pear also contains vitamin K which is good for brightening those dark circles that form under the eye and brightening dark spots around the body.

Natural sunscreen

Protect your skin from the sun and wind. A mixture of red earth (dug out from way deep inside the ground, where the sun and the oxygen can't reach it) and grease or tallow, rubbed on the skin, can be used as a natural sunscreen that will prevent sunburn. The red earth can also be used alone as a fine rouge.

Protect lips from the elements

Mint tea (made from Mentha arvensis) mixed with grease or tallow and rubbed on the lips, will keep your lips greasy and protect them from the sun and wind.

Skin cancer

To prevent skin cancer, if you work outside, wear sunscreen and perhaps a hat that shades your face.

If you get sunburned anyway

If you get sunburned anyway, rub yarrow tea on the sunburned skin. Yarrow tea will help soothe the pain and prevent peeling and blistering.

For skin dryness, rashes, breakouts and eczema

Evening primrose oil (from *Oenothera biennis*), which you can now buy from health-food stores, helps with skin dryness, rashes and eczema. It also works as a moisturizer. Taking it internally can also help to nourish your skin from the inside out.

Also, rubbing evening primrose oil mixed with vitamin E oil directly on the skin will help with rashes and skin breakouts.

For oily or dirty skin

Cake mud (now today's mud masks) on your skin and when you rinse it off, all the dirt, impurities and oil will also rinse off.

For tightening facial skin pores and a glowing face

Skunkbush liquid or tonic (from *Rhus aromatica*) makes a great astringent for cleaning out and tightening the pores in the face, leaving your face lustrous, and radiant. It tightens and firms the face and makes it look healthy and very smooth. The change can be amazing.

For detoxifying the skin

Juniper berries produce a detoxifying oil that is used even today as the active ingredient in some skin detoxification products.

For removal of oil, dirt, impurities and the opening of facial skin pores

Liquid or tonic from juniper berries also produce a stimulating, astringent that can be used to remove oil, dirt and impurities from facial skin. It opens blocked pores and keeps them clean and clear. Juniper enhances circulation and decreases swelling. This makes it an indispensable constituent in massage oil.

For poison ivy, bites and rashes.

Skunkbush tonic also helps to ease the pain of poison ivy, bites and rashes.

For warts

Green grass (picked in the spring) mixed with a little of your own spit and rubbed all over your warts will make the warts fall away.

Milky sap from milkweed (Asclepias species), rubbed unto warts will also make the warts fall off.

For acne

Apply a sudsy yucca (Yucca glauca) juice (made from yucca root), on the face to treat acne. Yucca root has plenty antioxidants including vitamin C and so protects, nourishes and soothes the skin. Yucca is also antibacterial, anti-inflammatory and detoxifying.

Teeth care

Natural teeth cleaning
Clean your teeth and gargle and rinse your mouth every day, in the morning upon waking up. You may clean your teeth with cooled cinders, charcoal.

Natural toothbrush/ tooth scrubber

You may use a single section of horsetail (Equisetum species) as tooth scrubber. The plant contains much silica, which helps grind off stuck-on food.

Natural toothpick

You may also use thorns from hawthorn trees (Crataegus species) as toothpicks.

Hair care/ hair issues

Best water for washing hair

Rainwater is the best water for washing and rinsing hair.

For faster hair growth

To make your hair grow faster, try braiding it regularly.

For incredibly shiny hair

To get your long hair to become superbly shiny, scrub sand into it and rinse it out really well. Rinse all the sand out. It works!

For repairing and restoring mature or damaged hair

Eat prickly pear and use the oil from its seeds to help strengthen hair. Prickly pear oil is rich in vitamin E and contains many fatty acids and proteins. This makes it a great remedy for mature and damaged hair. Its constituent oleic and linoleic fatty acids also help moisturize, soften and condition the hair.

For moisturizing, softening hair

Use agave (the tequila plant, a desert plant). The sugars in agave (that keeps the desert plant hydrated) bond with the internal proteins in the hair to add elasticity, strength and resiliency, and elasticity to hair.

For well-moisturized, shiny hair

Also, beaver oil rubbed into the hair, will moisturize the hair and give the hair a great shine.

For healthy, thick and strong hair

Liquid from boiled sweetgrass (bachuate, Hierchloe odorata) is a great after-shampoo rinse. It also makes hair to become healthy and thick.

Consuming the entrails and innards of animals, especially the stomach, (which contain the most protein), will help your hair to grow thick and strong.

For eliminating hair lice

Rinsing your hair with liquid from boiled greasewood (*Cercocarpus ledifolius*), also referred to as mountain mahogany) will work against lice.

For eliminating gray hair

Sage (*Artemesia* species) and iron, boiled together, is good for darkening gray hair and eyebrows (by the way, your gray roots won't show). This natural solution is obviously better than exposing yourself to the chemicals in modern-day dyes.

Baldness cure – for growing your hair back

Yucca (*Yucca glauca*). If you keep applying a sudsy yucca (Yucca glauca) tea (made from yucca root that was split with the grain and not across it), you will cure your baldness and your hair will grow back. But you must begin this treatment as soon as you notice balding. The sooner the better. In any event, give it a try now and see what happens.

White Prairieclover (*Dalea candida*). The Keres Pueblo Indians used this plant as a dermatological aid. An infusion of the roots of the plant was used as a hair wash to prevent hair loss.

Cosmetics

Rouge and face lifter

Red earth (that has not been exposed to the sun), as already mentioned, can be used alone as a fine rouge. It also acts as a face lifter and can make one look healthier and younger.

Eye-brow care

Charcoal may be used for darkening eye-brows to black. Elderberries may be used to shade eye-brows to blue, while juneberries may be used to shade eye-brows to purple (but note that juneberries stain). Grass may be used to make green eye-brow shades, while goldenrod flowers may be used to make golden yellow eye-brow shades.

Managing smells

Creating nice smells

Put some flowers (e.g. roses) in a bowl and close to you. From time to time, run your hands through the flower petals to stir the smell and enjoy the fragrance. You will feel better. This is what is called aromatherapy. Also, try burning some sweet pine, sage, or sweetgrass on a wood burning stove around your house. The fragrance is awesome and it is cleansing.

Masking foot odor

Try soaking your feet in cool mint tea for some time. Soak them two times a week for three weeks. It'll make the odor go away. Or you could try sage and sweet cedar. Flat sage (Artemisia ludoviciana) works against odors. Combine the sweet cedar (Juniperus scopulorum) with the sage, boil it, combine it in a container with clay to make mud and sit on a chair with both your feet placed inside the container of mud, for at least an hour or more. When you eventually scrub off the mud off your feet, all the dirt and odors on your feet will come off along with the mud. Sweet pine and sage both draw out toxins, dirt and smells and replace them with their own pleasant fragrance.

Masking body odor

Canadian thistles (Cirsium species) work against body odor. Just make tea out of the thistles and dash the tea on your armpits, then wash and dash and wash and dash and wash and dash until that area feels and smells clean. That'll do the trick. The odor will be gone.

Masking mouth odor

A little fresh mint will conquer mouth odor. So, try some mint tea! You may also chew on some fresh rose petals. That, also helps with mouth odor.

Longevity

How to stay young despite your age

Longevity and staying young is all about your attitude. It's all about how you think, the thoughts you allow in your head. Do not think or act old, and you won't be old. It's as simple as that. Also laugh as often as you can. Eat smart. Pray. And stay busy. You'll end up not even remembering to think or act old. This is the secret to longevity and remaining young forever.

CHAPTER 8: NATIVE AMERICAN HERBAL SECRETS FOR LOVE, PASSION, FLIRTING, APHRODISIACS, GETTING PREGNANT OR BUILDING A LONG-LASTING MARRIAGE

Native Americans have long been known to possess some herbal secrets for sparking love and passion and keeping that fire burning. Here are a few secrets you may put to use:

For flirting and attracting love

Elkweed, red root (*Ceanothus velutinus*). Try elkweed if you seek love. Just rub some dried elkweed leaves on your hands and a rub bit of it too on the person you wish to attract. That's all you have to do. And shortly thereafter, your love interest will surely find you wherever you are and start laying on the moves real thick. Honeymoons have been known to follow some of these elkweed-powder-fueled meets. You will be amazed at the wonders that will surely follow. This a very powerful herbal remedy, indeed! People become obsessed with you when you wear it. Elkweed also charms married couples to be attracted, affectionate, and committed to each other.

Aphrodisiacs

Wild onions (*Allium species*). If a little innocent flirting bores you and you wish to speed things up and move things to a higher, faster level, then you should mix clear pine sap with wild onions (Allium species) and eat the mixture. But be warned you'll get so hot, you might end up needing a fire truck to hose you down with "cooling-off water". That's how strong this special mixture can be. This is a very strong aphrodisiac. It may also help with impotence.

New England aster or Michaelmas daisy (*Symphyotrichum novae-angliae*). The Iroquois also used this plant as a "love medicine".

Vine Maple (*Acer circinatum*). Branches of this plant were used by the women of the Native American tribe, the Karok, as a "love medicine".

Northern Maidenhair (*Adiantum pedatum*). The Iroquois, used an infusion of this plant to induce vomiting as a remedy for love medicine.

Tall Thimbleweed (*Anemone virginiana*) The Iroquois used an infusion of the stems and roots of this plant as a love medicine for both males and females.

***Apiaceae Angelica* sp**. The Native American tribe, the Lolahnkok, used this plant as a love medicine. They rubbed the plant on the neck and hands of a girl to make her acquiesce and give in to love.

Spreading   Dogbane   (*Apocynum androsaemifolium*).
Warning: all the parts of this plant are poisonous. This plant should be handled and used with great

caution and only under the supervision of a licensed doctor. Nevertheless, the Native American tribe, the Okanagan Indians, are reported to have used this plant as a love medicine. They supposedly chewed the leaves and swallowed the pulp and the juice or they smoked the dried leaves of the plant as an aphrodisiac. These are all dangerous uses of this plant.

Yellow Pond Lily (*Nuphar sp.*). The Abnaki Indians used the Yellow Pond Lily as a love medicine and an aphrodisiac.

Yerba Buena (*Clinopodium douglasii*). The Karok used this plant as love medicine. An infusion of the leaves of this plant was taken as an aphrodisiac.

Longbract Frog Orchid (*Coeloglossum viride*). The Ojibwa Indians have used this plant as a love medicine. The plant was surreptitiously put inside another's food to act as an aphrodisiac. This was considered a bad use of the plant. And of course such conduct today would be against the law!

Canadian Lousewort (*Pedicularis canadensis*). This was another plant that the Ojibwa Indians put to use as a love medicine. The root of this plant was finely cut and was supposed to be surreptitiously put inside a strained love interest's food to act as an aphrodisiac and to cause the love interest to stop being quarrelsome and difficult and instead to become more loving and to become lovers again with their partner. The purpose was to promote and protect marriages and healthy relationships. But this plant was often misused in ways that would, today, be considered to be against the law and unacceptable.

Poison Hemlock (*Conium maculatum*). The poison hemlock is a highly poisonous plant which is poisonous to all mammals. You may recall that this is the plant that caused the deaths of Socrates, Theramenes and Phocion. Poisoning from this plant can result from either consumption, skin contact, or inhalation. Nevertheless, it has been reported that the Native American tribe, the Klallam Indians, put this plant to use as a love medicine. When a woman rubs the roots of this plant on her body, it is supposed to attract the attention of her male love interest to her.

Sacred Thornapple (*Datura wrightii*). The sacred thornapple is a poisonous plant. All of its parts contain hazardous levels of anticholinergic tropane alkaloids. This may cause death if consumed by humans, pets or livestock. In addition, it is now illegal in some places to sell, buy or cultivate this plant and other Datura plants. However, we note that the Costanoan Indians of California have used this plant as a love medicine. The seeds of this plant are mixed with tobacco and smoked for its aphrodisiac effect.

Tuliptree (*Liriodendron tulipifera*). The Rappahannock Indians used parts of this tree as a love medicine. The green bark of the tree was chewed raw as a sex invigorant. As at date, there are no known hazards of this tree.

For reversing impotence

Wild onions (*Allium species*). Eating clear pine sap mixed with a little wild onion will resolve that problem for you.

Quinine (*Cinchona calisaya*). Cherokee Indians used this plant as a reproductive aid. An infusion of the plant has been taken to cure impotence.

Rosy Pussytoes (*Antennaria rosea*). The Okanagan-Colville Indians used this plant as a reproductive aid. The leaves were masticated and ingested by men to increase their virility.

Alabama Supplejack (*Berchemia scandens*). The Houma Indians put this plant to use as a reproductive aid. A decoction of the bark and leaf has been ingested to cure male impotence and loss of libido in females.

For getting pregnant

Wild onions (*Allium species*). To get pregnant, try eating wild onions. Alternatively, you can eat foods like soy, which mimics estrogen. Also pray to get pregnant. Alternatively, you can build a small fire, throw in some sage and sweet pine incense into that fire. Then stand over the fire with your legs spread across and over the fire. Then hold your skirt, blouse or dress in a way that will trap the smoke from the fire underneath that garment and all round your waist region. Let that incense smoke swirl underneath your garment, around your legs and up towards your waist region. This works. But you must believe that it will work before you try it.

White Ash (*Fraxinus Americana*). The Iroquois Indians used this plant as a reproductive aid. Compound decoction of the plant's bark and roots were ingested to encourage pregnancy.

Kanawao (*Broussaisia argute*). Hawaiians used this plant as a reproductive aid. Eating the fruit with baked eggs was supposed to aid conception in barren women.

Golden Tickseed (*Coreopsis tinctoria*). The Zuni Indians used this plant as a reproductive aid. An infusion of the whole plant (with the exception of the root) is ingested by women who want to have female babies.

Bladder Seaweed (*Halosaccion glandiforme*). This plant has been used as a reproductive aid by the Nitinaht Indians. Newly-wed Nitinaht Indian women who wanted their first baby to be a boy chewed on sacs of this plant.

Bigseed Biscuitroot (*Lomatium macrocarpum*). The Thompson Indians have used this plant as a reproductive aid for elderly couples. The roots are consumed by elderly couples to aid them to conceive.

For preventing pregnancy (contraceptive)

Native Americans used various herbs made into infusions or teas and drunk (by the women) as contraceptives to prevent pregnancy. Some of these herbs include the following:

Saskatoon serviceberry (*Amelanchier alnifolia*). The Okanagan-Colville burnt branches of this plant, then boiled the ashes in water and drank the liquid to prevent getting pregnant. Also, the Thompsons made and drank tea from the fruit and leaves of the same plant for the same purpose.

Indian Paintbrush (*Castilleja affinis*). A decoction of this plant was ingested by the Tewa and Hopi Native American tribes in order to prevent pregnancy.

White Turtlehead (*Chelone glabra*). The leaves from this plant were made into a tea by the Malecite and Micmac Native American tribes to prevent pregnancy.

One seed juniper (*Juniperus monosperma*). The leaves of this plant were used to prepare an infusion/tea which the women of the Zuni Native American tribe drank to prevent conception. The Shoshone also made their own tea with the berries from this plant and drank the tea, every morning for 3 consecutive days, to prevent conception.

Bitter Cherry (*Prunus emarginata*) The Quinalt, Skokomish, Lummi and Skagit Native American tribes used this plant as a contraceptive. They allowed the wood to rot, then soaked the wood in hot water and drank the resulting liquid to prevent getting pregnant.

California False Hellebore (*Veratrum californicum*). The Shoshone, Paiute and the Washo native American tribes made tea from the root of this plant which was drunk by both women and men to prevent conception. But this false hellebore tea was thought to cause permanent sterility in some cases.

Western Gromwell (*Lithospermum ruderale*) works as a contraceptive. But be very careful with this plant. It is so strong and if overused, can permanently prevent pregnancy (cause sterility). An infusion of the roots of this plant ingested daily for 6 months would cause permanent sterility.

Spreading Dogbane (*Apocynum androsaemifolium*). Warning: all the parts of this plant are poisonous. This plant should be handled and used with great caution and only under the supervision of a licensed doctor. Nevertheless, the Okanagan Indians, are reported to have used this plant as a love medicine. They boiled the roots of this plant in water and drank the liquid once a week so as to prevent pregnancy. This is an unsafe use of this plant as such a use can cause dangerous side-effects.

For broken hearts

Elkweed, red root (*Ceanothus velutinus*). Use elkweed for a broken heart. Your love will come back to you. But if your lover still leaves you, then let the person go. That person is not meant for you. Look for someone else who is truly meant for you.

For a stable and long-lasting marriage

Elkweed, red root (*Ceanothus velutinus*). Again, use elkweed occasionally.

Satinleaf (*Chrysophyllum oliviforme*). The Seminole Indians used this plant as a love medicine. A decoction of wood ashes from this plant is put on the tongue. Supposedly this strengthens your marriage and cleanses your body.

Southern Bayberry (*Morella cerifera*). The Seminole Indians also used this plant as a love medicine. A decoction of wood ashes from this plant is also put on the tongue. And supposedly this also strengthens your marriage and cleanses your body.

Cardinalflower (*Lobelia cardinalis*). The Meskwaki Indians used this plant as a love medicine and to prevent divorce. The roots of this plant were ground and used in preparing food to be eaten together by a couple in a strained marriage or relationship. After eating such food, the ground roots of this plant used to make the food was supposed to cause the couple to end their quarrel or misunderstanding, forgive each other and make up, thus forestalling divorce.

Great Blue Lobelia (*Lobelia siphilitica*).
The Meskwaki Indians used this plant as a love medicine and as a remedy against divorce. The roots of this plant were finely chopped and consumed by a couple in a strained marriage or relationship in order to renew their love to each other and to avert divorce.

American Ginseng (*Panax quinquefolius*). The Seminole Indians used this plant as a love medicine and as a post-divorce remedy. An ex-husband rubs the plant on his body and clothes in order to get back his divorced wife.

Coastal Plain Willow (*Salix caroliniana*). The Seminole Indians used this plant as a love medicine. The bark of the tree was used as a medicine to supposedly prevent adultery.

Purple Meadowrue (*Thalictrum dasycarpum*). The Meskwaki Indians used this plant as a love medicine to settle and reunite a quarrelsome couple.

Native American socialization. But in addition to all of the above, there were some fundamental principles that Native Americans understood and were socialized into which were aimed at promoting long-lasting marriages. They understood and taught that when you get married, your spouse becomes your lover, friend and sibling, and vice versa. Each of these roles carries special responsibilities which you and your spouse must respect and carry out.

At times your spouse will need you as a friend (will need you as a sounding board, will need your advice, will need your companionship, etc.). At other times your spouse will need you as a sibling (will need your comfort, forgiveness, prayers, etc.). And of course, your spouse is your lover and needs you as a lover, frequently expressed in words, acts and, of course, love making.

A married couple needs to respect and lovingly perform all of these three roles satisfactorily to each other in order to have a long-lasting marriage or to at least have a chance at a long-lasting marriage.

CHAPTER 9: SPECIAL NATIVE AMERICAN HERBAL REMEDIES FOR MAKING YOURSELF FLU-PROOF

Viruses are the causes of colds and flu. And viruses are pretty darn tough agents! They cannot be killed by pharmaceutical drugs, chemicals or herbal compounds. The only way to manage and survive a viral attack is to motivate your body's own immune defense system to kick into gear and resist and fight off the virus. That process will involve at least three fundamental steps as follows. You must:

(i) Eject the invader (the virus)
(ii) Nurture and sustain the tissue that was attacked or via which the virus was able to take root (in the case of the flu, that would be the respiratory system).
(iii) Provide support to your immune system to enable it to forestall a relapse.

Herbs that alleviate fever, congestion, cough and other symptoms can help you to manage the side-effects and the opportunistic health issues that come along with the infection, while your immune system moves the infecting virus out of your system.

1. Eject the virus

When you notice the signs and symptoms of flu and cold, quickly attack them with natural remedies so that you may recover within 24 hours. To achieve this and as time is of the essence, you have to be proactive.

Osha root (Ligusticum porteri). Start with this herb. It is a potent North American herb that's widely considered as very effective against respiratory infections. Osha is also called "mountain ginseng", "mountain carrot" or "bear root". The plant comes from the parsley family (includes dill and carrot) and can be found mostly in the high altitudes of the Rocky mountain states and the Southwest. In modern herbology, osha is trusted as a first line defense against respiratory infections.

Osha is bitter to the taste, although the root has a numbing, soothing effect on sore throats. Osha is also an expectorant. It is also used to treat coughs, colds, early-stage tonsillitis, bronchial pneumonia, flu and fever.

An in vitro study carried out at Texas A & M University in 2016 confirmed that osha has potential as an immunomodulator and that it is protective against oxidative cellular damage. Osha can be taken along with Echinacea to support the white blood cells in their resistance against infection.

Today, osha can be purchased in herbal stores (either as dried, powdered roots, or as decoctions or other liquid formulations, or in capsules or as the whole plant. Osha is contraindicated for those who are pregnant, nursing or that have acute inflammation of the kidney.

2. Nurture and sustain your respiratory system

If you are already down with the flu, the following herb will help you recover faster. If you desire to shorten your recovery time from the flu, then the following herb might be your remedy.

Andrographis (*Andrographis paniculata*). This herb has been and is used in Native American, Chinese and Ayurveda herbalism as effective against upper respiratory infections (e.g. bronchitis or the flu, along with the associated headache, fever and body ache), sinusitis, tonsillitis, laryngopharyngitis, and general inflammation. Andrographis is also used for alleviating and reducing the symptoms and duration of colds.

Since the 1970s, over 676 studies on andrographis have been published confirming the effectiveness of andrographis in the treatment of colds. In one study, the severity of the symptoms of cold experienced by the study participants (those who had cold), had significantly reduced by the fourth day following treatment with andrographis. In another study, after five days of 85mg of andrographis extract taken three times a day, 68% of the study participants reported that they had recovered completely from their cold, compared to 36% from the placebo group. 55% of the treated group considered their colds as uncharacteristically mild and they took less time away from work. In short, the scientific consensus appears to be that andrographis is safe and beneficial for the treatment of the symptoms of acute respiratory tract infection and for the shortening of recovery time from infection.

3. Prevent a relapse

If, however, you are a victim of recurring flu attacks, you will need a longer-term strategy to help you out. You will need to consider using Isatis root and/or Lomatium root.

Isatis root (*Isatis tinctoria*). This herb is of the cabbage family. It is a broad-spectrum antimicrobial used primarily to reduce fever. Recent studies show that components from isatis root are immunostimulating. A 2015 in vitro study published in the Journal of Ethnopharmacology found a constituent in isatis root that also has anti-flu-virus properties. Isatis root may be used alone to treat the flu or in combination with another herb (astragalus root). In fact, isatis root and astragalus root combine well for the treatment of the flu and many other physiological conditions. These two herbs also combine well to fortify the lungs.

So, to treat the flu, you may use isatis root alone for no more than a total of 20 grams per day. Or you may use isatis root in combination with astragalus root, still for no more than 20 grams per day, spread through the day. Both herbs are safe.

Lomatium root (*Lomatium dissectum*). Lomatium root is also worth considering. Once widely considered to be a powerful healing agent by Native Americans, it was used extensively to treat influenza. Recently, lomatium is again being used as an effective remedy in the treatment of upper respiratory tract infection (both viral and bacterial). Most people use lomatium in tincture at a dose of 60–90 drops, 3 to 4 times per day. But you need to know that it can cause a measles-like rash in some people.

CHAPTER 10: HOW TO HANDLE. PREPARE AND STORE HERBS FOR GOOD HEALTH AND WELLNESS

Native Americans lived close to the earth and so they intimately interacted and understood their environment more fully and thoroughly than we can imagine. To them, their food, medicine and life as they knew it, came from their environment. Under their circumstances, they were compelled to learn the mysteries of the earth and to use the secrets they learned to protect their health and enhance their lives.

To the Native Americans good health is not necessarily a specific medication, rather it is an unending cycle that involves the medication (herb), the disease, the patient, the community, the earth, faith, discovery and gratitude, all molded together in a didactic experience from which they observed and learned. And they gave thanks for each and every healing remedy that nature revealed to them.

So, the Native American concept of disease or ill health was not one of precision, since good health to them was more or less like a continuum, made up of what life and living was also entirely made up of.

It was modernity that brought medications that are able to fight disease with microscopic precision. These modern pharmaceuticals characteristically zero in on and disrupt or end certain specific genetic, cellular or organic function/s in order to end the enduring process of a particular disease.

However, often these microscopically precise processes come with side effects that sometimes feel worse than the underlying disease. Besides, modern medicine often only treats symptoms with precision, without activating the body's innate capacity to heal itself and without operating holistically and synergistically (principles around which Native American medicine basically revolved).

The point is that there are no new health issues as such. This is because hundreds of years ago the humans that lived at that time (including the Native Americans) had, more or less, faced the same health problems, issues and concerns that we face today. And very importantly, over a slow and deliberate process of trial and error, they had discovered effective and enduring solutions that still heal and protect good health up to today.

Indeed, it is difficult to believe (but it is true) that ancient natural remedies that were developed and perfected from eons ago, can today, not only effectively complement modern medicine, but in some cases, even exceed and beat the abilities of modern medicine. And luckily all of these natural treasures have been bequeathed to us and are available to any of us who wishes to source their good health from the greatest power and source of good health (Mother Nature). In short, we ought to be thankful for the many natural and effective healing secrets that the Native Americans bequeathed to us.

Now, here is some advice on how to handle some of these treasures that were bequeathed to us by the Native Americans and mother nature.

Harvesting

Herbs should be harvested when the plant has enough foliage to support growth and when the oils responsible for their taste and fragrance are at their peak. The right timing is a great factor when it comes to harvesting. You can use either a pruner or sharp knife to cut plants for harvesting. Cut annual herbs between 50 and 75 percent and 1/3 of perennial plants for easy regrowth.

Harvesting should be done early in the morning. Also harvest before the herbs begin to flower. And ensure that the herbs to be harvested have not been previously sprayed with pesticide as that might make the herbs unfit for consumption.

Drying

The primitive way of preserving herbs is the use of low heat or drying by air. Wash herbs gently and carefully dry them using paper towels after harvesting. Remove any damaged/dead material and tie in loose bunches for easy circulation of air. Bunches can be put in paper bags with punched holes for ventilation. The bags serve as protection from contamination and dust. Bunches can be hung in a shed, garage, barn or any dry, warm and ventilated place.

Herbs of short stems can be dried using a tray. Arrange herbs in it and place out in the sun or in any well-ventilated place. You may need to turn the leaves from time to time to ensure complete drying.

Dried herbs can be removed and packaged in tight containers out of the sun in cool places. To retain their flavor, avoid crushing the leaves during packaging. The flavor of herbs can be retained for about a year if properly stored.

Seeds of herbs can also be dried by cutting their stems with seed heads before they turn brown. They should be gathered in bunches and hung upside down in well-ventilated places. Shake the seed from their seed heads, carefully separating them from their capsules. Seeds can be blown to remove chaffs and debris. Seeds can then be stored in tight containers. While seeds may take longer to dry than leaves, ensure that they're properly dried before storage to prevent them from getting moldy.

Preparing

Native Americans had great faith in their herbs, as they used all parts of plants, prepared in various ways. Herb usage varied, however, according to the different tribes, with each tribe and each healer having its or his own unique recipes and method of preparation.

Sometimes, the herbs were smoked or burned (to be inhaled), or taken as tinctures (mixed with alcohol) or made into salves by combining them with fats of animals or made into infusions or decoctions.

Traditionally, they could be chewed to extract the oil and apply to affected areas. Interestingly, for certain desired therapeutic effects, some healing ceremonies called for patients to be burned with the smoldering branches of some herbs.

However, the most prevalent herbal preparations weren't so exotic. The Native Americans, in fact, prepared many herbs in much the same way as today's herbalists do. There are indeed various ways of preparing herbs, but below are the most common methods for simple use:

Teas and infusions

Teas are also called infusions. They are prepared by steeping bark, seeds and leaves in hot water, straining the bark, seeds or leaves and drinking the remaining liquid. Sometimes the liquid is also applied to bruises, burns, sprains and cuts.

To prepare tea, drop a teaspoonful or two teaspoons of dried herbs and fresh herbs respectively in a boiling water (one cup) to infuse for 15 minutes and strain using filter. Drink when cool immediately as it will lose it potency after few hours.

To make stronger infusions, double the above measurements, but note that exceeding this can lead to health complications.

Decoctions

This is the method used for harder plant parts. To prepare a decoction, an ounce or two ounces of dried herbs or fresh herbs respectively are put in cool water (a pint), in a pot and put to the boil for an hour. Strain the content and allow to cool before drinking. Alternatively, you can add it to your bathwater to bathe with or you can soak towels in the solution to use for massaging. The decoction is most effective if drunk immediately or put in a tight container and stored in the refrigerator for no more than 24 hours, maximum.

Poultices

Poultices are mostly used for exterior problems, such as skin irritations, wounds, swellings, sores, sprains, bruises or arthritis, etc. A poultice is made up of a pulp that is created by mashing herbs to a paste or by tenderizing dry herbs by boiling them for about ten to fifteen minutes. Another way to make a poultice is to do it the way Native Americans often did it and that is to
masticate the herb into a pulp (without swallowing the liquid) and then applying the pulp/paste onto the skin.

The poultice needs to be placed directly on the area being treated, that is directly on top of the skin or putting it between two gauzes or thin cloths and then placing it on the area being treated and securing it in place.

Note that some individuals are allergic to certain herbs, and that areas of the skin being treated with poultices may show signs of irritation or stress. These could be signs that an allergic reaction is occurring and, in that case, the treatment should be discontinued immediately and medical attention sought.

Herbal remedies and children

Before using herbal remedies with your kids, consult your physician or any experienced native healer because children react differently to herbs than adults.

The following recommended herbal dosage for infants, kids and teens should be adhered to:

From 0 to 1 year, 1/20 of adult dosage. For 2&3 years, 1/10 of adult dosage. From 3 &4 years, 1/5 of adult dosage. From 5&6 years, 3/10 of adult dosage. From 7&8 years, 2/5 of adult dosage. For 9&10 years, ½ of adult dosage. For 11&12 years, 3/5 of adult dosage. For 13&14 years, 4/5 of adult dosage. while 15 years and above can take the full adult dosage.

Here are additional guidelines for gathering, drying and storing herbs:

Additional guidelines for gathering

Note the following precautions while gathering herbs:
•Ask, do any laws, including local laws, allow or prohibit the picking of plants or the picking of this plant?
•Ensure that where you are planning to harvest your herb is not a high-pollution area (e.g. a busy highway) or you may pick up polluted herbs.
•Ensure that you pick only the right herb to avoid poisoning. Be sure of what you are doing.
•Don't over harvest or damage the remaining herbs while harvesting.

•Respect the environment as the Native Americans did.

Additional guidelines for drying

Note the following guidelines for drying herbs:
• Unless herbs are properly dried and stored, they can easily lose their potency.
• To dry fresh leaves, separate them from their stems and spread them on flat/clean surfaces to dry.
• To dry bulky plants, hang them from a line in a dry airy area such as an attic or a warm basement.
• To prevent flies or insects from perching on the herbs you are drying, you may want to cover the herbs with a thin layer of cloth.
• The duration required for drying a specific herb depends on the drying environment and the herb itself but the shorter the drying duration, the better.
• One week is a good drying duration for herbs.
• Herbs have dried sufficiently, when they have become breakable, while still retaining their aroma.
• To dry roots, wash them thoroughly before drying. And roots dry longer than leaves and flowers.
• To wash and clean roots properly before drying them, hand-brush the roots and use a pressure hose to flush out the dirt. Remember that rinsing alone will not properly remove the dirt.
• Average drying duration for roots is 3 weeks.
• To dry roots string them or just lay them out.
• To check whether a large sample root is dry, cut it in half and check the center.
• To dry herbs, lay them out in dry, shaded, airy areas.
• Do not dry your herbs on newspaper prints or wire screens.

• Do not wash flowers or leaves before drying. Instead shake them vigorously to get any dust or bugs off.
• To dry leaves, you may scatter them loosely on flat, dry, clean surfaces or you may tie the leaves in 2 inch (or less) bundles at the base of their stems.
• To dry barks, you may scrape off the exterior of the bark if necessary.
• Any plant part that is brittle to the touch is already dry.

Storing

Note the following guidelines for storing herbs:
• Store dried roots in metal, ceramic or dark glass containers, covered with tight lids.
• While storing herbs, avoid excess heat and light in order to prevent the destruction of some essential properties in the herbs.
• Store dry herbs in food-grade plastic containers or any such containers that omit moisture and oxygen. This will help to preserve the potency and quality of the preserved herb.
• Label your stored herb containers with dates and location information.
• Do not crush or break herbs. Compared to uncut, whole herbs, crushed or broken herbs are quicker to lose their essential properties and value.

www.ingramcontent.com/pod-product-compliance
Lightning Source LLC
Chambersburg PA
CBHW061336250726
48657CB00004B/1189